The Death of Eric Garner

How Did Almost Everyone Get it So Wrong?

2nd Edition

James Crothers

Copyright © 2019 James Crothers

All rights reserved.

ISBN-9781095673966

PREFACE

As a scientist, I was disturbed by the way in which evidence was carelessly, and perhaps with strong bias, misrepresented in news reports about the deadly arrest of Eric Garner in the Staten Island borough of New York City on July 17, 2014. Almost all reporters characterized his death as a vicious "chokehold killing" by one policeman.

Science has a strong commitment to the careful, truthful presentation of evidence with unbiased, rational, knowledgeable analysis. Interpretation of how Eric Garner died should not be influenced by political leanings or the pursuit of some larger social objective, but be determined strictly by analysis of the evidence in that case.

I spent about thirty months trying to get various journalists, news organizations, and politicians to consider an alternative (physiologist's) analysis of what was revealed in the widely seen video shot by Ramsey Orta, but kept hitting a brick wall. After a book by Matt Taibbi and a decision by the New

York City Civilian Complaint Review Board, both in late 2017, reasserted widely held misperceptions, I finally resorted to a belated presentation of the alternative analysis in the form of this book, now in a revised and updated second edition.

This analysis is neither a politically left-wing view of Garner's arrest as racist brutality nor a right-wing "Breitbart" view that the police did nothing wrong. In this interpretation of the evidence, Eric Garner is still considered to have died because he was mishandled by the police. However, he was not killed by a chokehold.

Of course, Garner should not have died in that incident, as no one should die for just being arrested, regardless of the reason for the arrest. While a correct interpretation of just how Garner died does not change the fact that the NYPD was responsible for his death, it should greatly affect the legal — and social — aftermath. To understand how he died, and why a police officer was not indicted for a chokehold killing, read on...

— James Crothers

CONTENTS

Chapter		Page
1	What happened?	1
2	What is compressive asphyxia?	14
3	The fatal outcome	38
4	A digression about jumping to conclusions	45
5	The beginning of the misinterpretation	48
6	The medical examiners	54
7	A digression about chokeholds	76
8	The journalists	84
9	The DA and the grand jury	131
10	The Department of Justice	163
11	The CCRB and the NYPD	185
	Postscript	195

Chapter 1

What happened?

In 2014, action by the New York City Police Department against sellers of smuggled cigarettes that evade New York taxes and are often sold singly as "loosies" was intensified on orders from the Chief of the Department, Philip Banks III, as reported by John Marzulli, Rocco Parascandola, and Thomas Tracy in the N.Y. Daily News, Aug. 7, 2014. Whatever we may think of New York's high cigarette taxes, they were not set by the NYPD, nor were its patrol officers responsible for the city's policy, often called "broken windows," of increased enforcement of laws against minor crimes.

Eric Garner was a distinctively tall and large man who had been arrested multiple times on various charges, including selling loosies, in the Tompkinsville neighborhood of Staten Island and was well known to the police. He was apparently identified, or sufficiently described, in some "311 calls" as engaged in such illegal cigarette sales on July 17. It was also reported that a police lieutenant called the 120th Precinct that day and, based on his own observations, asked it to send officers to Tompkinsville Park, where Garner regularly sold cigarettes illegally. Justin Damico and Daniel Pantaleo were the ones who were sent.

Details about just how the decision was made to arrest Garner have not been fully publicized. I have not seen any reports saying that the NYPD knew, at that time, the full extent of Garner's cigarette-smuggling operation, described in Matt Taibbi's book, *I Can't Breathe: A Killing on Bay Street*, published in late 2017. According to Taibbi's research, that operation involved Garner regularly paying drivers to bring cartons of cigarettes, from locations with low cigarette taxes, for him to resell as packs or loosies at a modest profit on the streets in Staten Island. Even without that full knowledge, those checking the identification and police record of the person described either in the 311 calls or by the lieutenant would surely have found that he was out on bail and scheduled for a court appearance a few weeks later (reported on SILive.com, July 18, 2014). The NYPD could have justified the arrest of Garner on this day as a *revocation of bail*, not requiring the arresting officers actually to have seen him committing a crime just before the arrest, but based on complaints or observations by others. Even Taibbi, though his book was sympathetic to Garner and strongly critical of the NYPD, conceded that, based on the evidence he had seen, the two policemen seemed to be acting under orders and couldn't just let Garner go if they did observe him selling loosies.

Damico and Pantaleo drove to Tompkinsville Park, as directed. Whether or not they actually saw Garner sell loosies at that time, they got out of their car and moved to arrest him on the sidewalk. Witnesses at the scene thought police had come in response to a brief fight that Garner had just broken up and were surprised that the focus was, instead, on Garner. Ramsey Orta, a friend of Garner, then used his cell phone to start a video recording of the encounter. It is difficult to overstate how important that video is for understanding what subsequently happened to Garner. It is equally difficult to overstate the importance of the failure of almost everyone who viewed the video either to study it carefully enough or to have the necessary knowledge to interpret what it showed. Careful, repeated viewings of that video are crucial for the description, here, of what occurred during the attempted arrest.

The officers spent at least five minutes trying to convince Garner to accept a peaceful arrest. They

What happened?

can be seen already standing on either side of him at the beginning of the video, so we don't know how much earlier the encounter began. The officers were speaking quietly and we have difficulty hearing most of what they said, but they had certainly told him they were placing him under arrest, since we hear Orta describe them as "tryin' to lock somebody up for breakin' up a fight," and we hear Damico say, "We can do this the easy way or the hard way." Garner repeatedly refused to submit.

The officers finally gave up on the effort to get Garner simply to walk to their car and get in ("the easy way"). With back-up officers arriving, Pantaleo began an attempt (still peaceful) to handcuff Garner, first gesturing to him to put his hands behind his back (probably also speaking a command that we can't hear), then grabbing his right wrist from behind. Garner yanked his right arm upward out of Pantaleo's hand and pulled his left arm up, resisting Damico's efforts to grab that arm from the front. The officers then moved to the standard next step, wrestling him down, as any policemen would do to someone who yanks his arms out of their hands while they try to handcuff him during an arrest.

The video showed Pantaleo trying to use a maneuver that police call a "seatbelt" at the beginning of the takedown, in this case bringing his right arm up under Garner's right armpit and angling his left arm down over Garner's left shoulder (that arm suggesting the shoulder strap of a car's seatbelt). Applied in that way, it might have been intended to twist Garner down sideways by pulling up on the right shoulder and pushing down on the left. Garner was tall enough and massive enough that Pantaleo had difficulty getting his left forearm very far over the left shoulder. Nevertheless, the positioning of his right arm under the right armpit distinguishes this kind of hold from an intentional chokehold.

What happened?

The two men spun around, with the newly arrived officers ineffectively trying to grab Garner's arms or torso. After Pantaleo and Garner bumped into a storefront window, Pantaleo finally began to pull Garner down to his left, away from the window. Virtually all published accounts of this takedown describe Garner as being pulled down with a chokehold, although Pantaleo's right arm was still under Garner's right armpit. They were facing away from the camera then, but we can see that, during the hard pull, Pantaleo's left forearm rose to a position such that his hand and wrist, not visible to us, would have come up to the front of Garner's neck. With the force needed to pull Garner away from the window and down, that hand and wrist were likely to have caused bruising of neck muscles, later described by the New York City medical examiner.

When Garner started falling to his left, he lifted his right arm, reached it across his body to brace his fall, and twisted his body leftward, so Pantaleo lost the right half of the seatbelt hold, his arm no longer wedged under the armpit. About five seconds after the start of the takedown, Garner came down on his left thigh. He then rolled to a crouch, lurching forward on hands and knees, bringing Pantaleo along on his back. Pantaleo's left arm remained next to Garner's neck and we can briefly see, through a gap between other officers, Pantaleo's right arm near Garner's right side, but nowhere near his neck. Pantaleo's right hand then moved to grab his left hand, *over* Garner's right shoulder, in an apparent effort to maintain some kind of hold, as Garner was still resisting restraint and no other officer had yet gotten a grip on Garner. With that hold, Pantaleo's arms became looped in a way that they would not slip up past Garner's head, displaying, at the end of the seventh second of the takedown, the *first appearance* of a possible chokehold.

What happened?

They then rolled over, both ending with their right sides on the pavement. At this time, ten seconds into the takedown, Garner can be considered to have stopped resisting, his right shoulder against the pavement, his right arm extended in front of him, and his left arm being brought toward his back by another officer. His legs were already turned toward the prone position, both knees on the pavement, with his belly beginning to be squeezed against the pavement.

At the start of the twelfth second, Pantaleo began raising himself to a kneeling position on the pavement with his arms still looped around Garner's neck, providing widely publicized images interpreted by almost everyone as obviously showing a chokehold, though the left forearm could have been pressing up against Garner's chin, maintaining a *restraining* hold. Before the end of the twelfth second, Pantaleo released his right hand's grip of his left hand and extended his right hand to hold

Garner's right arm. About fifteen seconds after the start of the takedown and five seconds after Garner was finally down on his right side, Pantaleo's left arm slipped off Garner's neck as the other officers rolled Garner's torso into the fully prone position.

As Garner's belly became more severely compressed against the pavement, he began saying, "I can't breathe," and Pantaleo shifted his attention to holding Garner's head, left ear against the pavement, face to his right. Garner's right arm was then brought toward his back, by another officer, for handcuffing. With Garner remaining in the prone position during the handcuffing effort, his "I can't breathe" protests continued, gradually fading to inaudibility, so the exact number of those protests is difficult to count, but often reported to be eleven. Garner eventually went unconscious and limp.

Because the NYC medical examiner reported that the arm around the neck left no damage to any part of Garner's airway (including trachea, larynx, and the delicate hyoid bone that is commonly broken in cases of actual strangulation), the restriction of Garner's breathing when he was actually saying "I can't breathe" and going unconscious was not directly caused by that arm. According to the evidence, the only injury that can be fairly conclusively attributed to that arm was bruising, or slight hemorrhaging, to neck muscles around the airway, most likely to have happened during the sharp yank away from the window, when Pantaleo's arms were not in the position of a chokehold.

It is still *possible* that Pantaleo's arm caused some restriction of Garner's breathing before it was eventually released. However, with no *evidence* that Garner's breathing *was* restricted during that time, together with the facts that Garner was conscious and speaking when the arm was released and he was only evidently having difficulty breathing during the subsequent prone restraint, a conclusion that the arm around his neck *acted as* a chokehold is not supported.

Since the medical examiner said that the bruising was not detected during the initial external examination, it would not have been noticed at all if there had been no autopsy. If the officers had rolled Garner onto his belly for only a few seconds to bring his right arm behind his back, then quickly rolled him back onto his right side to complete the handcuffing, Garner would simply have been secured and taken to the police station, alive, with *no detected injury* other than possible minor scrapes on his arms or legs. Conversely, imagine that, when the back-up officers arrived, the whole group wrestled Garner down by grabbing his arms, legs, and torso, with no one even touching his neck. If they then continued exactly as in the actual incident, restraining Garner belly-down on the sidewalk for just as long, he would have been asphyxiated exactly as he actually was, by a phenomenon called *compressive asphyxia*.

Chapter 2

What is compressive asphyxia?

Compressive asphyxia occurs when various kinds of pressure on the torso result in severe restriction of the volume to which the lungs can be expanded. The mechanism most often involves compression of the abdomen, the lower part of the torso, squeezing abdominal contents (the "guts") up against the diaphragm, keeping the diaphragm from being lowered enough to allow adequate intake of air. Inhaling does involve some expansion of the rib cage, but the main mechanism by which we expand the lungs to inhale air is the lowering of the diaphragm, causing some outward expansion of the belly as the diaphragm pushes downward on the guts. By placing a hand over our belly and watching it during a deep breath, we can see and feel that expansion. If expansion of the belly is prevented — or, worse, the belly is *compressed* — by an outside force, lowering of the diaphragm may be restricted, possibly so much that not enough air is inhaled to replace oxygen the body is using.

Serious crushing accidents can greatly compress the rib cage, breaking some ribs. Moderate compression of the chest can occur if a heavy man is sitting or kneeling on the upper back of someone restrained in a prone position. But, the rib cage is more than strong enough to prevent significant compression of the *chest* during prone restraint when there is almost no force other than the detainee's own weight compressing his torso. The larger a detainee's belly, the more seriously his *abdomen* will be compressed during prone restraint, pushing the diaphragm upward and increasing the likelihood, *as well as the rapidity*, of deadly asphyxiation. Furthermore, someone in the prone position with his arms secured behind his back cannot push those arms against the ground to decrease the pressure on his belly.

Such asphyxia occurring to people being restrained in the prone position on pavement, ground, or floor tends to be called "positional asphyxia" or "restraint-related positional asphyxia." The prone position can also be called "face down," so information about restraint in this position may include a warning that breathing can be impaired if the mouth and nose are directly against the surface on which a person is being held. Such impairment is *obstructive* and is distinct from the *compressive* asphyxia that may be occurring at the same time. Compressive asphyxia does not block the respiratory airways, so air can flow freely in and out, but the *volume of air per breath* is greatly limited by restricted expansion of the lungs. Thus, someone experiencing this condition may be able to make short statements — like "I can't breathe" — when the small breaths are exhaled.

The maker of a restraining device called "The WRAP," the major portion of which is wrapped around someone's legs while he is still in the prone position *after* being handcuffed (thus extending the duration of prone restraint), warned on its web site to "make sure the subject can breathe." The NYPD officers arresting Garner were also quite likely to have been taught to "make sure the subject can breathe" while he is in prone restraint. They seemed to feel sure that Garner *could* breathe because he was repeatedly speaking and his face was being positioned to the side by Pantaleo. The fact that Garner's *words* were clearly heard (until his voice became too weak) was consistent with his mouth not being blocked. Several officers were later quoted as saying, "If he can speak, he can breathe," to explain why Garner's words were not taken seriously. The officers did not seem to have been trained to understand compressive asphyxia well enough to know how someone can be speaking repeatedly *while* suffering this kind of asphyxiation. Knowledge of the "dead space" helps us understand how.

The respiratory tract has extensively branching air passages which, below the *larynx* (voice box), are collectively called the "bronchial tree." They resemble an upside-down tree with the *trachea* as its trunk, the two *primary bronchi* branching left and right from it, then much additional branching resulting in smaller and smaller *bronchioles* — ultimately tens of millions of *terminal bronchioles*, each carrying air to and from a cluster of microscopically small, extremely thin-walled sacs called *alveoli*. It is through those very thin walls that inhaled oxygen reaching the alveolar spaces can diffuse quickly into the tiniest blood vessels (*capillaries*) in the alveolar walls. The air passages (including mouth, nose, and pharynx, as well as the bronchial tree) constitute what is called a "dead space," because their thicker walls and limited blood flow don't allow significant gas exchange with the blood stream and they have a total air space of about 150 ml in a person of average size. Thus, about the last 150 ml of each inhalation don't reach the alveoli and remain in the dead space, their oxygen then leaving the respiratory tract, unused, with the next exhalation. (What constitutes the dead space is a bit more complicated, as one can learn from a physiology textbook, or from various web sites discussing "respiratory dead space," but the simpler description of it, as the total space in air passages leading to the alveoli, will suffice here.)

When we have been sitting quietly for a while, doing what is called "resting breathing" with a fairly low oxygen need, we tend to inhale a volume of air about three times the volume of the dead space, usually with fifteen or fewer breaths per minute. In this condition, the first two thirds of inhaled air reach the alveoli and the last third stays in the dead space until exhaled. When we are more active, we inhale not only more frequently, but a larger volume of air per breath.

Without knowledge of the dead space, one might think that rapid small breaths could add up to the same air intake per minute as less frequent larger breaths. If the small breaths are 200 ml × 45 per minute and the larger breaths are 600 ml × 15 per minute, both might seem to provide 9000 ml of air per minute. However, with the dead space of 150 ml subtracted *from each breath*, the useful fresh air reaching alveoli per minute would be 50 ml × 45 = 2250 ml and 450 ml × 15 = 6750 ml, the rapid small breaths being considerably worse than the less frequent larger breaths. In a situation in which someone needs to have about 6000 ml of fresh air per minute reaching his alveoli to replace oxygen being used by his body, those rapid small breaths would result in a net loss of oxygen from his body, a condition called *hypoxia*, which will continue to worsen if the lungs cannot be more fully expanded. With those small breaths, though only 50 ml of *fresh* air would reach alveoli per breath, 200 ml of air would pass through the *voice box* with each exhalation (mostly fresh air that didn't reach alveoli with the previous inhalation), allowing repeated speech that might seem inconsistent with asphyxiation.

If the volume of air in each inhalation is *no larger* than the dead space, virtually none of the fresh air will reach alveoli, so virtually none of its oxygen will get into the bloodstream. During each small exhalation, "spent" air (low in oxygen and high in carbon dioxide) will leave the alveoli, going into the dead space, and that spent air will be the *only* air going back into the alveoli with the next small inhalation. As this "trapped" air repeatedly goes back and forth between alveoli and the dead space, there will be a steady decrease in its oxygen and an increase in its carbon dioxide. In terms of respiratory function, inhaling only the dead-space volume would be no better than not breathing at all. Yet, repeated short statements would still be possible until increasing hypoxia leads to unconsciousness. Garner had a type of body in which compression of the guts against the diaphragm would be quite extreme during prone restraint and he went unconscious quickly enough that each of his breaths during that restraint must have been little larger than his dead space.

In 2013, Robert Ethan Saylor, a 26-year-old man with Down syndrome died that way in Maryland when sheriff's deputies, moonlighting as mall security officers, were trying to remove him from a movie theater. He had simply wanted to stay and watch a movie a second time without having a second ticket. With Down syndrome, he had childlike characteristics, didn't understand why he couldn't just stay in the theater, and was having what his caretaker later characterized as a "tantrum," fighting against the deputies. They eventually wrestled him into a prone position on the floor to handcuff him.

In early reports of the incident, Saylor's obesity, a typical physical trait of Down syndrome, was described as preventing the deputies from bringing his arms close enough together behind his back for a single pair of handcuffs to connect his wrists. Very sadly, during the extra time the deputies spent trying to chain three pairs of handcuffs together, Saylor reportedly called for his mother with his small breaths before going unconscious and limp. One deputy later described Saylor's skin as having "turned gray."

The deputies were reported to have tried to revive him with CPR (Cardio-Pulmonary Resuscitation), but I have not found a news article that indicated whether they performed the pulmonary ("mouth-to-mouth") part of CPR or only the cardio (chest-pumping) part. The latter is commonly used by itself, but is not helpful for someone who has just been asphyxiated if, as in Garner's case, his heart keeps beating for minutes longer. Saylor, like

Garner, needed to get *enough* air into his lungs quickly — over and over — but I doubt that the deputies understood his need, any more than the NYPD officers understood what Garner needed. The deputies in the Saylor case were not indicted by a grand jury, possibly because the jury determined that the deputies had not been taught an adequate understanding either of Down syndrome or of compressive asphyxia, and that they considered prone positioning for handcuffing to be standard procedure.

In 2014, James Greer was subjected to a field sobriety test after a traffic stop in Hayward, CA. Apparently deciding that Greer was not fully compliant during the test, police wrestled him into a prone position long enough to handcuff him and then, as he continued struggling, to secure The WRAP around his legs. He went unconscious and could not be revived, his lips described as having "turned blue." A color change of various body parts to bluish or grayish is called *cyanosis*, an indication of serious hypoxia because blood is bright red when fully oxygenated, but dark purple when very poorly oxygenated. As in the Saylor case, news reports did not specify exactly what techniques were used in the attempt to revive Greer.

The web site for The WRAP showed a picture demonstrating someone in the prone position, already handcuffed behind his back, with The WRAP ready to be secured around his legs. Its larger piece goes around the knees, requiring three straps to be buckled, while a separate, smaller tie goes around the ankles, but the site made no mention of a danger of compressive asphyxia if the time in prone restraint is greatly extended by securing of The WRAP.

A medical examiner decided, from evidence of some PCP in Greer's body, that he died from "over-exertion under the influence of PCP." As a physiologist, I consider the medical examiner to have missed the obvious: 1) Greer had a very large belly, seen in police body-cam video, making him *certain* to suffer compressive asphyxia if held belly-down on the pavement too long, 2) he spent a long time in that prone restraint, partly because of the use of The WRAP, and 3) his lips had turned blue during that restraint.

This type of death will typically leave no evidence of the cause detectable in autopsy, so medical examiners limiting themselves to studying the body may have trouble determining the cause. If someone is simply rolled onto his belly, then restrained in that position with his guts (soft tissue) being squeezed up against his diaphragm, there may be no bruising to the skin of the torso, no cracked ribs, no damage to intercostal tissue, and no injury to internal organs, such as a ruptured spleen. Medical examiners need to look beyond autopsy evidence, taking into consideration all available evidence of the circumstances leading up to the death, and must have an adequate understanding of compressive asphyxia to be able to consider it a reasonable, even likely, explanation. This kind of death almost certainly occurs much more commonly than revealed in official cause-of-death records.

In 2017, police had a warrant for the arrest of Humberto Martinez in Pittsburg, CA. A video showed him jumping out of a car and running into a house, with police in close pursuit. Martinez reportedly engaged in vigorous physical resistance, with use of a Taser against him having little effect. An early news report of the incident quoted a witness inside the house as saying that Martinez "turned blue" after he was finally wrestled down and held in prone position on the floor. The video of Martinez running into the house showed him having a large belly that would have been compressed during prone restraint. He did not recover from that restraint and died.

While there is an important issue of police not being adequately trained to handle people who behave somewhat differently from the majority of the population because of conditions like Down syndrome, that issue is outside the scope of this book. The point to be made here is that all those who sometimes need to restrain another person must be trained to have a better understanding of compressive asphyxia, especially that a detainee's belly size and total body weight can greatly increase the deadly danger of prone restraint.

Some asserted, as did Donna Lieberman, executive director of the NY Civil Liberties Union, that Garner's arrest, takedown, and death for a minor infraction like selling loosies would never happen to a white person (reported by City & State editor, Gerson Borrero, May 6, 2015). Her assertion was a falsehood irresponsibly inflaming racial tensions. People resisting arrest are usually wrestled down, no matter what their race is. Compressive asphyxia during restraint by law enforcement officers also happens without regard to the race of the detainee and happens too often, with police departments being inexcusably slow to gain adequate knowledge of the phenomenon to pass on to their patrol officers. A decision by the Ninth Circuit Federal Court in a 2003 case (Drummond v. City of Anaheim) included the statement, "The compression asphyxia that resulted appears with unfortunate frequency in the reported decisions of the federal courts, and presumably occurs with even greater frequency on the street."

Garner, Saylor, Greer, and Martinez all died in essentially the same way. Only one of them, Garner, was black. Garner did not die "because he was black," any more than Saylor, Greer, and Martinez died because they were not black. Furthermore, the "minor infractions" are a side issue. Garner did not *die* for "selling loosies." Greer did not *die* because of "a sobriety test." Saylor did not *die* because "he wanted to see a movie again without a second ticket." They *died* because those restraining them were not taught an adequate understanding of compressive asphyxia. Those who directly caused these deaths almost certainly did not intend to kill someone with the prone restraint and almost certainly did not know that they *were* killing someone while they were using that restraint. The phenomenon of compressive asphyxia needs to be much better taught to police, sheriff's deputies, state troopers, prison guards, mental hospital attendants, and any whose occupations may sometimes require them to restrain others.

Compressive asphyxia can occur in other positions and even without any physical force exerted by another person. In Oakland, CA, in 2015, Richard Linyard sprinted away from police trying to arrest him on an outstanding warrant, then hid by wedging himself, upright, into a narrow gap between two buildings. When police finally found him, nearly an hour later, and pulled him out, he had suffered asphyxiation and could not be revived.

Although Linyard was thinner than Garner, body-cam video showed him, before he turned and ran, having a moderately bulging belly that would have been compressed into his torso when he squeezed into that gap, which police measured as only $11^1/_2$ inches wide. After having sprinted some distance, he would have felt rather "winded," and was likely to have thought that the rapid small breaths he was taking while wedged into that narrow space were simply the panting he would expect to do after such exertion, probably thinking, "I just need to catch my breath; I'll be OK." He would not have understood that the volume of those breaths was not enough larger than his dead space to meet his oxygen need after a strenuous run and he would have gone progressively hypoxic until he passed out. Once he was unconscious, he could not extricate himself to stop the ultimately fatal depletion of his oxygen.

How did Garner, unlike Linyard, so quickly realize that he "couldn't breathe" adequately? Garner was quite large and had been for many years. He was likely to have experienced the phenomenon before, in more familiar ways, such as waking up at night, gasping for air, finding himself belly-down in the bed, and realizing that he had to roll off his belly to breathe adequately. When he was rolled onto his belly on July 17, 2014, Garner probably knew, immediately, how seriously his breathing would be limited and tried, with his very small breaths, to tell the police. They, inadequately trained, mistook the fact that he *was speaking* as more important than *what* he was saying.

The Linyard example illustrates that compressive asphyxia may occur without actions that are violent or brutal and, thus, may be done by someone with no intent even to hurt, much less kill, another person. With Garner, those actions began after he was down on the sidewalk and they consisted of police simply rolling him into the prone position and keeping him in that position for too long as they handcuffed him. Ironically, the actions of police during *the takedown* (with an arm on his neck), seen by nearly everyone as a vicious, deadly assault, did almost no harm to him.

Prone positioning for handcuffing is a long established practice and is done for good reason. Someone in that position has almost no ability to bite, to strike with his arms, or to kick with his legs. Nevertheless, such restraint is potentially deadly, as already extensively described here. A slender person might suffer compressive asphyxia in prone restraint only if he experiences the additional compressive force of someone kneeling or sitting on his back, but a person with a sizable belly and large body mass can experience such asphyxia if he is just restrained by his arms and legs in the prone position, with his own body weight compressing his larger abdominal contents against his diaphragm.

Individual policemen are likely to have restrained many people in the prone position without a deadly result, because those who are most likely to require such restraint would tend to be younger and fitter, possibly thinking they can fight back or successfully flee. Much more likely to submit to peaceful arrest are those who are somewhat older, and overweight or obese. With relatively few of the latter group resisting arrest and with about a half million patrol law-enforcement officers in the United States, most of those officers have not learned, directly from their own experience, the deadly danger of prone restraint for people who are larger and heavier. The officers need to learn in their training, so they don't have to find out *by actually killing someone,* though, unfortunately, even when such deaths do occur, the cause is often misunderstood. With men, as opposed to women, being the ones who deposit most excess body fat in their bellies, and with the number of people falling into the categories of overweight or obese increasing in the United States, there must be tens of millions of men in this country who could die just as Garner, Saylor, Greer, and Martinez died.

In the San Francisco Bay area, news reports have characterized several recent in-custody deaths following use of stun guns as "Taser deaths." Though the events were very briefly described, all seemed to involve prone restraint *after* use of the Taser, with the arrestee "becoming unresponsive" *during that restraint.* Arresting officers, police chiefs, sheriffs, reporters, attorneys, and medical examiners all seem not to have considered the possibility of compressive asphyxia in these cases, with the visibly obvious stun gun capturing their attention. The danger of prone positioning, especially for the heavier men who resist restraint, *must* become much more widely understood.

The N.Y. Times quoted NYPD guidelines about the danger of positional asphyxia as saying, "As soon as the subject is handcuffed, get him off his stomach. Turn him on his side or place him in a seated position." Unfortunately, "as soon as the subject is handcuffed" may not be soon enough, since obesity can greatly shorten the time in which deadly asphyxiation can occur, while also lengthening the time in prone restraint by increasing the difficulty of getting the detainee's wrists together behind his back. In addition, the guidelines seem not to have explained the respiratory dead space and, thus, the phenomenon of being able to speak repeatedly while being asphyxiated.

Breathing through an external tube, as in snorkeling, increases the dead space by the volume of that tube. Snorkelers, when they start to feel a bit "breathless," should take larger, not just more frequent, breaths to compensate for a larger dead space. A recent spate of deaths among snorkelers in Hawaiian coastal waters called attention to a new device, a full-face snorkel mask, which may enlarge the dead space, increasing the portion of inhaled air that is merely "spent air" from the previous exhalation. Some newer snorkel designs, perhaps not yet widely used, mostly separate the pathways for inhaled and exhaled air, greatly reducing expansion of the dead space. This may seem a bit off the topic of "compressive" asphyxia, but it emphasizes the importance of inhaling a large enough volume of fresh air *in excess of* the dead-space volume.

An interesting comparison can be made between deadly compressive asphyxia and the life-saving Heimlich maneuver. "The Heimlich" is designed to compress the thoracic space, increasing air pressure under an object stuck at the top of the airway, pushing the object out. Standing behind someone who is choking, you would properly apply the maneuver by wrapping your arms around his torso, under his arms, and positioning a clenched fist over his *belly* (not on his chest). Your forearms would just touch the lowest ribs. With your other hand over your clenched fist, helping to increase force, you would apply *brief, strong* pressure on both the belly (with your fist) and the lowest ribs (with your forearms) by pulling backward very quickly and forcefully. This action sharply increases pressure within the thoracic space — therefore within the blocked airway — by forcing abdominal contents up against the diaphragm, pushing it upward, and by pressing the lower ribs inward. If the person being choked is in a chair (since the choking object is most often a piece of food) and can't stand up, pressure of your forearms against the victim's sides may be somewhat limited by a chair back, so sharp, hard squeezing of the belly may be most important. The crucial difference between this maneuver and compressive asphyxia is the duration. *Brief* squeezing of the abdomen to push the diaphragm upward may save a life, while *sustained* squeezing of the abdomen can be deadly.

Chapter 3

The fatal outcome

When Garner went unconscious, the police could feel that he had gone limp and would have realized that something was wrong. Since they had incorrectly deduced, from his repeated statements, that he *could* breathe, they were puzzled and did not guess that they had asphyxiated him. They rolled him onto his side, much too late, but they attempted no kind of resuscitation. Some onlookers were heard asking, "Why is nobody doing CPR?" An officer replied that Garner was breathing.

Garner had apparently become hypoxic enough to be adversely affected beyond mere unconsciousness. The portion of his brain (the respiratory center in the medulla) that controls involuntary breathing was likely to have become less effective, but still able to direct weak, fitful breathing, like an extreme version of sleep apnea, with frequent long gaps between breaths. His sporadic breathing at that time turned out to be inadequate, so his hypoxia — and, thus, his breathing — continued to worsen, though more gradually than during the prone restraint.

What Garner needed immediately at that time was the "pulmonary" part of CPR — air repeatedly blown into his lungs. Recently, more and more people are thinking of CPR as *only* chest pumping, perhaps appropriate immediately after someone has suffered a heart attack or other cardiac arrest, but Garner's heart was apparently still beating quite well, as the heart can continue beating with no signaling from the brain. Not until he was in the ambulance being taken to the hospital did his heart stop, most likely because his oxygen level had then dropped too low for cardiac muscle cells to make enough of the cellular "energy molecule," ATP, needed for all muscle cells to contract.

Another bystander's cell-phone video began after the end of the Orta video, several minutes before an ambulance arrived with emergency medical technicians (EMTs), one of whom then checked Garner's vital signs, apparently satisfied by a normal pulse. That video shows that Garner was still handcuffed while being examined by the EMT, who should, therefore, have realized that the police had been handling Garner while he was still conscious. But, the EMT seemed to make no effort to ask the police what they had been doing to Garner *when he went unconscious*. Such a question should be standard procedure for EMTs, since it can elicit important clues to the medical condition facing them. If the police had been asked such a question, they should have said that Garner was being handcuffed, prone on the sidewalk, when he went unconscious and limp. The police should even have provided that information to the EMTs without being asked — along with the fact that Garner had been repeatedly saying, "I can't breathe." If the EMTs had found that someone with Garner's body type had gone unconscious during prone restraint, they should have considered asphyxia to be the likeliest possibility. But, were *they* adequately trained to understand *compressive* asphyxia?

Did the EMTs look at Garner's fingernails? Although people with lighter skin may be easily seen as turning bluish or grayish when they become extremely hypoxic, that cyanotic change might not be seen over most of the body of someone with darker skin. Almost all of us (except a rare few with genetic albinism) have some level of the dark brown protein, melanin, in our skin, the amount of which can be increased with exposure to sunlight ("tanning"). However, skin beneath the fingernails usually lacks melanin, even in dark-skinned people, leaving the fingernail beds appearing a light pink when blood is properly oxygenated. Garner's fingernails should have appeared bluish or grayish when he was seriously hypoxic. Did the EMTs have a simple *pulse oximeter* that could have revealed serious hypoxia if clamped on one of Garner's fingers? If the EMTs could have determined that Garner was likely to have been asphyxiated, they should have begun getting air into his lungs, possibly immediately by mouth-to-mouth breathing, switching to a hand-squeezed ventilating bag using pure oxygen from their portable tank as soon as that was ready.

While police clearly need to acquire a more complete understanding of compressive asphyxia caused by prone restraint, EMTs and paramedics ought to be thoroughly trained to understand such a medical emergency. However, this review of the responses of emergency medical personnel is not meant to place principal blame on them. Although Garner might have been resuscitated, his actual asphyxiation by prone restraint and the failure of any policemen to understand what they were doing, and had done, to him should still be considered the main causes of his death.

An EMT or paramedic called in, saying that Garner's heart stopped while he was in the ambulance. Some reporters and commentators called it a "heart attack," a term that should be used to refer to damage in a portion of heart muscle caused by blockage, or severe restriction, of blood flow through a coronary artery to that part of the heart, something that could have been seen as mainly the result of *pre-existing* cardiovascular disease. However, the medical examiner reported no evidence of such damage, so the stopping of Garner's heart was almost certainly due to deepening hypoxia throughout his whole body — caused by *asphyxiation in this incident.* Although he was only officially pronounced dead at the hospital, surely after attempts to revive him, the stopping of his heart in the ambulance might reasonably be considered the time of his death.

Chapter 4

A digression about jumping to conclusions

When I was in my childhood, many movies and television dramas presented stories set in the 19th-century western American frontier. A fairly common story line involved someone suspected of a serious crime in a small town, being held in a jail cell in the local sheriff's office and awaiting transport to a larger town with a courthouse where a trial could be held. A growing crowd of angry townspeople was gathering on the street, threatening to storm the small jail and drag the suspect out to be hanged, shot, or beaten to death. The angry mob felt absolutely sure of the suspect's guilt and didn't want to wait for the legal process to run its proper course.

These dramas would continue in various ways, sometimes with the suspect killed by the mob, followed by later discovery that someone else actually committed the crime. Sometimes, the "good" sheriff would prevail, protecting the suspect and guaranteeing him his right to a trial (in which he still could be convicted, but legally). I came to realize that we were being given civics lessons in the importance of the often slow legal process and the need to refrain from jumping to conclusions.

In high school, I considered journalism as one possible career and thought that I perceived journalistic ethics to bar the practice of "convicting someone in the press" before there was an actual conviction in a court of law. While the publications we commonly call "tabloids" or "rags" frequently engage in that practice, it seemed to me that the more respectable journalists were expected to refrain from doing it.

A digression about jumping to conclusions

Reading news coverage of Garner's death, I was troubled that virtually the entire "respectable" journalistic profession had "convicted" officer Pantaleo of a chokehold killing before he could "have his day in court." Much worse, that "conviction" continued even *after* he had his day in court — *after* a grand jury decided that the evidence did not even support indictment, much less conviction, for a chokehold killing.

One of the important rights the American Civil Liberties Union has long sought to uphold is a suspect's right to be presumed innocent until convicted in court. Yet, I have seen no sign of the ACLU defending Pantaleo's right, either directly or by chastising journalists for "convicting" him in the press.

We all need more of those old civics lessons.

Chapter 5

The beginning of the misinterpretation

Those who have watched movies and television shows for decades have seen many examples of fictional policemen wrestling down a resisting suspect during a fictional arrest and may have seen, more recently, such takedowns by real policemen in "reality shows" that follow police who are on their rounds or responding to reports of crimes. Even if takedowns looked rough, we would accept them as routine procedure, perhaps partly because it seemed that "bad guys" were being wrestled down and partly because the takedowns that we saw rarely (if ever) resulted in death, real or acted.

The beginning of the misinterpretation

In real-life situations, police who are arresting someone will typically tell him that he is being placed under arrest and tell him to put his hands behind his back. If he doesn't comply within about two seconds, they will grab his arms. If he then yanks his arms out of their hands, they will immediately start wrestling him down. The whole process could take fewer than ten seconds, with the police being considered to have acted properly. Even some bruises or a scraped knee experienced by the person being arrested would be considered unremarkable and quite acceptable.

However, millions who viewed the Orta video, knowing in advance that Garner's arrest ended with his death, reading that the arrest involved selling "loosies," and seeing that a black man was being arrested by white policemen, interpreted the entire event through a "lens of outrage." The fact that he was being arrested at all was called inexcusable. Most people simply did not *see* that he refused to put his arms behind his back when directed to do so and then yanked his arms out of the officers' hands as they tried to handcuff him. Garner was not deemed to deserve being wrestled down because he was not being violent (or even threatening violence) against police. N.Y. Times editors later described the takedown as a "lethal assault."

Unfortunately, the Daily News first posted a version of the video having much of the initial verbal interaction with Garner deleted, giving many an impression of undue haste in the decision to wrestle him down. The Boston Globe editors later (Dec. 4, 2014) described it as an example of "police officers who make no effort to resolve situations peacefully," even though police in this case actually spent a *very* unusually long time (at least five minutes, and probably more) trying to accomplish the arrest as peacefully as possible. Furthermore, most people, not knowing that the officers were sent to that location, by their superiors, to deal with the "problem" of illegal cigarette sales, initially guessed that Damico and Pantaleo spontaneously chose to harass a randomly encountered black man over a minor infraction.

From the very start, the Orta video was described, in numerous web postings, as showing Garner being killed by a chokehold. With careful, *knowledgeable* study of the video, one can discern the compressive asphyxia that was not literally *seen* by anyone, but the public perception was obviously limited to the very visible arm around the neck.

The video does not show Garner's death, but everything in it was interpreted with the advance knowledge of that end result, making it quite gut-wrenching to watch *and hear*. Donna Lieberman (quoted by James Queally, July 19, 2014, in The Chicago Tribune) said, "It's painful and horrifying to watch the video knowing throughout what the end is." It would seem that most people, with that emotional response, shied away from watching multiple times — and more carefully — so they clung to poorly perceived or poorly remembered initial impressions of the video.

One of the almost immediate, and commonly repeated, misrepresentations of the video was that the "I can't breathe" statements came *during* the alleged chokehold. It is possible that people's quick interpretation of a chokehold killing led their minds to create false memories that fit and supported that conclusion. A day after the incident, Jumaane Williams, a New York City councilman, issued a statement that included, "... the video of an unarmed man screaming in a chokehold that he can't breathe disgusts me." Rev. Al Sharpton was repeatedly quoted as having said, at Garner's funeral, "... a man in your arm saying, 'I can't breathe' .... When does your morality kick in? You don't need no cultural orientation to stop choking a man saying, 'I can't breathe.'"

Hardly anyone had any knowledge of compressive asphyxia, so the arm around the neck seemed the only possible cause of death. It *must* have been a chokehold, which *must* have been causing Garner to say that he couldn't breathe. Although one news article two days after Garner's death quoted an unnamed source in the medical examiner's office as saying that no damage to any part of Garner's airway was found, the report may have been noticed by too few people who, in turn, failed to perceive what it meant for the possible role of a chokehold in the restriction of Garner's breathing when his neck was no longer being touched by Pantaleo's arm. People did not consider the problem of how that arm could have been causing asphyxiation during the prone restraint — when the "I can't breathe" statements are actually heard — and the faulty connection between the alleged chokehold and the asphyxiation became quickly and very firmly established.

Chapter 6

The medical examiners

The brief press release on Aug. 1, 2014, from Dr. Barbara Sampson, NYC Chief Medical Examiner since Feb., 2013, stated that Garner died from "compression of the neck (choke hold), chest compression and prone positioning during physical restraint by police," with acute and chronic bronchial asthma, obesity, and hypertensive cardiovascular disease as contributing factors. It was not explicitly stated that the order of principal causes indicated order of importance, but virtually everyone interpreted the meaning to be that a chokehold was the main cause of death. After reviewing the autopsy results on Sept. 19, 2014, Dr. Michael Baden (a retired medical examiner doing consulting work) stepped out of Dr. Sampson's office and, on the sidewalk, quickly told reporters (AP, Sept. 19, 2014), "Compression of the neck that prevents breathing trumps everything else as cause of death."

I suspect that both medical examiners were working with a professional bias in favor of autopsy as the "gold standard" for determining cause of death. Both would have been medically trained (MD), with additional post-doctoral training in the specialty of forensic pathology. Essentially, they were specialized in performing and interpreting autopsies. Both may have considered a cell-phone video shot by a bystander to be peripheral evidence that just seemed to support autopsy evidence of a chokehold. They apparently didn't study the video carefully enough to perceive what it revealed about the precise *timing* of events.

Dr. Baden might have had another bias. He was hired by lawyers for Garner's family right after a police union spokesman said that a chokehold was not used on Garner. Jillian Jorgensen wrote (Observer, Sept. 19, 2014) that Dr. Baden was accompanied by a lawyer for Garner's family when he spoke to reporters right after emerging from Dr. Sampson's office. That family is well known to have concentrated its anger against Pantaleo and was surely wanting Dr. Baden to confirm that Pantaleo's arm around the neck was mainly, if not solely, responsible for Garner's death. Maintenance of that focused blame for more than three years was reported by Benjamin Mueller, who wrote (N.Y. Times, Sept. 8, 2017), "Mr. Garner's widow, Esaw Snipes, said ... it was most important to her family that Officer Pantaleo face criminal charges. Mr. Garner's mother, Gwen Carr ... said the Police Department should fire Officer Pantaleo and he should serve prison time."

Jorgensen reported that, in the same sidewalk interview, Baden also "said his review was not complete and would include referencing the autopsy report with video and eyewitness statements in an attempt to determine things like when the compression to Mr. Garner's neck occurred." Thus, it was irresponsible of him to tell reporters, "compression of the neck ... trumps everything else as cause of death," when he had yet to compare the autopsy evidence to video and eyewitness evidence.

The Orta video, not the autopsy, was actually the most important evidence in the Garner case. It provides crucial evidence that cannot be gleaned from an autopsy, the most important possibly being a precise timeline. The abstract of an article, "Asphyxial death during prone restraint revisited" (O'Halloran & Frank, *Am J Forensic Med Pathol.* Mar, 2000), stated, "Establishing a temporal association between the restraint and the sudden loss of consciousness/death is critical to making a correct determination of cause of death."

Only the video allows the time during which Pantaleo's arm was touching Garner's neck to be seen as separate from the subsequent time during which Garner was in a prone position on the sidewalk. Only the video enables us to perceive that all of his "I can't breathe" statements came while his belly was down on the sidewalk, with nobody touching his neck. Only the video enables us to hear his speech fading steadily to inaudibility just during the prone restraint. Only the video shows him going from conscious and speaking at the start of the prone restraint to unconscious and limp by the end of that restraint. The evidence that Pantaleo's arm left no damage to any part of Garner's airway and the lack of any evidence of Garner having difficulty breathing before he was rolled onto his belly not only make it impossible for that arm to have been the direct cause of Garner's restricted breathing *after* the neck hold was released, but also undermine a conclusion that the arm restricted Garner's breathing at any time *before* it was released. This paragraph describes the *timing problem,* which will be mentioned often in the chapters to come. Furthermore, only the video shows different kinds of contact with Garner's neck during the takedown, allowing reasonable guesses to be made about when, and how, the neck was most likely to have been bruised.

The NYC medical examiner seemed to overemphasize two kinds of autopsy evidence that only *suggest* a chokehold, with Dr. Baden later offering his enthusiastic support for the chokehold interpretation. Those two kinds of evidence are 1) bruising to neck muscles (*strap muscles*) on both sides of the airway, and 2) some petechial hemorrhaging in the eyes, often seen after — and often interpreted as caused by — strangulation. Both call for some detailed analysis.

All of us have experienced bruises — possibly many hundreds, depending on how rambunctious we were as children, the kinds of athletic activities in which we engaged, and how long we have lived, among other things. Something we know about our bruises is that almost all were caused by very brief contact between some part of our body and something (or someone) else. Most of us would be very unlikely to use the word "pressure" to describe the *brief impact* that usually causes a bruise. Choking someone to cause significant restriction of breathing would, in contrast, involve sustained pressure. Although such pressure may cause bruising, reasoning in the opposite direction — that bruising indicates sustained pressure — is not justified. That would be an example of what is commonly the first error of reasoning discussed during an academic course in logic: "if A, then B" does not necessarily mean that, "if B, then A."

The Orta video does not show Pantaleo's left arm squeezing on Garner's windpipe as the "seatbelt" hold was initially applied. After the two bumped into the storefront window, Pantaleo might have suddenly feared the danger of breaking the window, leaving sharp edges of glass that could slice into arteries, quickly causing fatal blood loss. He pulled very hard to bring Garner, and himself, down to his left, away from the window. The two of them were facing away from the camera at that time, but the position of the visible part of Pantaleo's left forearm suggests that his hand and wrist did go up to the front of Garner's neck as he pulled hard. All the motions of Garner and Pantaleo seen in the video, from the initiation of the "seatbelt" until Pantaleo released his arm fifteen seconds later, seem to show that by far the strongest force exerted by Pantaleo came when he yanked Garner away from the window, with a force that lasted about one second and would have been a somewhat sideways force, from Garner's right to his left. If the base of Pantaleo's thumb was on one side of Garner's airway and the radial bone of his forearm on the other side, with the bend of his wrist over the airway, the strap muscles on both sides of the airway could easily have been bruised with no detectable damage to the airway itself.

Spitz and Fisher's Medicolegal Investigation of Death, a 1300-page tome often described as "the Bible for forensic pathologists," describes a "bar arm" chokehold as a forearm going straight across the front of someone's neck, with the wrist pulled by the choker's other hand to increase the force of the arm on the front of the neck. Pantaleo's arms appeared that way in the eighth second of Garner's takedown and the NYC medical examiner seemed to interpret the bruising to Garner's strap muscles on *both sides* of his airway as caused by just such a chokehold. However, the same page in *Spitz* describes that chokehold as having the "potential for injury of the airway," including "laryngeal fractures." Since the strongest force exerted by Pantaleo seemed to be in the yank away from the window, when his left arm was not in the bar arm position — the bend of his wrist in front of the airway decreasing the force exerted on the larynx — the bruising on both sides without damage to the airway is more consistent with that *brief* yank away from the window, during the "seatbelt" maneuver, than it is with the later *apparent* chokehold.

After his right arm was no longer retained under Garner's right armpit, Pantaleo appeared to be just trying to regain some kind of hold until the other officers got control. He seemed to gain that hold — around Garner's neck — by the eighth second of the takedown. It is merely a *possibility* that some bruising occurred during the remaining eight seconds before Pantaleo released his left arm. However, since the only actual signs of Garner's difficulty breathing began when he was rolled into the prone position and the arm was no longer around his neck, the evidence does not support a conclusion that the same action that caused the bruising *also* caused restriction of breathing.

"Petechial hemorrhaging" is an expression many have heard in television shows in which an actor playing a medical examiner mentions it as evidence of strangulation when it is seen in the eyes. *Petechiae* (singular, *petechia*) are tiny specks of blood leaked from very small blood vessels, the smallest and weakest being the capillaries. The front of the eyeball is covered by an extremely thin, delicate, almost fully transparent tissue called the *conjunctiva*, in which capillaries have relatively little support from surrounding tissue and are rather susceptible to leakage if blood pressure within them rises too high. Outside the perimeter of the iris, the conjunctiva extends over some of the eyeball's white tissue, the *sclera*, providing a background against which even very small petechiae can be quite visible. Elevation of blood pressure in cranial veins, possibly caused by constriction of the jugular veins that carry blood away from the head through the neck, will necessarily raise pressure in the capillaries that drain into those veins, possibly causing petechial hemorrhaging in some parts of the head, most likely — and most easily seen — in the delicate conjunctiva. Strangling someone would almost necessarily constrict the jugular veins, so it is quite likely that, if someone has been strangled, petechiae would be seen in the eyes. However, one should not commit the previously mentioned error of logic by "reasoning" that, if petechiae are seen in the eyes, they must have resulted from strangulation.

In various web sites, one can read about petechiae and learn that petechial hemorrhaging in the head may have any of numerous non-fatal, even quite minor, causes that do not involve constriction of the neck. Some of those causes involve elevated pressure *within the torso*, sometimes in repeated spikes, as from bad coughing, or sometimes in a more sustained way, as during the action called "straining at the stool" when one is experiencing constipation. Increased pressure inside the torso necessarily raises the normally low pressure in the jugular veins and, thus, raises pressure in cranial capillaries without any constriction of the neck. Such increased pressure might have occurred to Garner some time before this encounter with police, or might have occurred as his abdomen was being compressed against the sidewalk and he was squeezing out his pleas for adequate breath. Even if the petechiae observed in Garner were caused by compression of his jugular veins during that encounter, rather than by elevated pressure in his torso, those veins are located toward the sides of the neck, so pressure on either of them during the takedown would not necessarily mean that there was also constriction of the airway.

A review article by Dr. Susan Ely and Dr. Charles Hirsch (*J Forensic Sci*, 2000), who were then working in the NYC Medical Examiner's Office, strongly made the point that petechiae in the eyes or face result not directly from asphyxiation, but from elevated pressure in cranial veins. In one test described by the article, human subjects displayed petechiae in their eyes after one minute of being held in a vertical upside-down position, raising pressure in cranial veins and capillaries without constriction of the neck and certainly without asphyxiation.

Though any bleeding (blood escaping from blood vessels) can be called *hemorrhage*, that word is usually used for serious bleeding that can result in significant blood loss from the circulatory system. A *bruise* involves very slight bleeding, in a region usually in and just under the skin, from numerous small blood vessels so close to each other that the visual appearance, to the naked eye, is a diffuse purplish discoloration. *Petechial hemorrhaging* is so called because, although it is very slight bleeding, it appears as distinctly separate specks of blood. The injury to Garner's strap muscles has been described either as bruising or as hemorrhaging. While the NYC medical examiners' full autopsy reports are not publicly released, Dr. Baden used the word "hemorrhages," which suggests the possibility of bleeding from some tiny tears in the muscles, leaving distinctly separate spots of bleeding. That appearance might be consistent with Pantaleo exerting a hard force that quickly moved the skin somewhat sideways against the underlying muscles, as during the sharp yank away from the storefront window. That could cause slight tearing of some muscle fibers, with the skin (moving with the arm) not showing any bruise detectable during external examination.

The notion that the arm around the neck restricted Garner's breathing is simply an inference from the bruising and petechial hemorrhaging, both of which could easily have resulted from causes unrelated to choking. The inference is overwhelmed by the facts that 1) there is no direct evidence that Garner's breathing was *actually* restricted while the arm was touching his neck, 2) Garner was conscious and speaking right after release of that arm, going unconscious and limp only during the prone restraint, 3) all the "I can't breathe" statements came during the prone restraint, after the arm was released, 4) his voice faded steadily to inaudibility during the prone restraint, consistent with depletion of his body's oxygen occurring during that time, 5) the arm left no damage to the airway to cause difficulty breathing during the time when asphyxiation was obviously happening, and 6) Garner's body type made it virtually certain that he *would* experience compressive asphyxia if held in the prone position on a solid, flat surface.

Both medical examiners used the words "chest compression" to characterize part of what happened to Garner. This wording suggests the possibility that neither of them understood compressive asphyxia well enough. The way it was experienced by Garner, it involved mainly compression of his belly, squeezing guts up against the diaphragm. "Chest compression" could have been intended to mean that, when the compressed guts push the diaphragm upward, the volume of the thoracic cavity would decrease. But, it seems quite clear from some of Dr. Baden's comments that he was referring to pressure directly exerted on the external surface of the chest, which would have been insignificant in the asphyxiation of Garner.

Dr. Baden seemed to realize that his hasty sidewalk statement blaming "compression of the neck" was not adequate to explain Garner's difficulty breathing during the prone restraint. He was seen, in a later interview on the Fox network, miming with his hands the way he thought officers were pressing down on Garner's back. He said, "There was pressure on the neck and pressure on the chest that interferes with the lungs expanding, and hands on the face and nose, so he couldn't breathe ...." He was quoted in the N.Y. Times as saying, "Obese people especially, lying face down, prone, are unable to breathe when enough pressure is put on their back. The pressure prevents the diaphragm from going up and down, and he can't inhale and exhale." Actually, direct pressure on the chest is likely to have far less effect on "up and down" movement of the diaphragm than does the squeezing of abdominal contents up against the diaphragm — for "obese people especially." Dr. Baden's statement also conflicted with the fact that Garner was repeatedly speaking during his asphyxiation, meaning that he *had to be* "inhaling and exhaling" — just not nearly enough air per breath.

Finally, the description of "hands on the face and nose" was blatantly false, since the Orta video shows no such thing and Garner's repeated words had to come from an uncovered mouth.

Some researchers have subjected volunteers who are young and healthy, and are not overweight, to experimental prone restraint, then presented their results as proving that this kind of restraint does not significantly restrict breathing. However, anesthesiologists, who must maintain constant monitoring of the vital signs — including oxygen level — of surgical patients, became aware, decades ago, of seriously restricted breathing in patients undergoing the kinds of surgery (e.g., spinal surgery) requiring prone positioning. It was found that, for patients with protruding bellies, some kind of support method is needed that allows the belly to hang below the level of the chest and pelvis, so abdominal contents are not squeezed up against the diaphragm. There are some support apparatuses that are patented, manufactured, and marketed to achieve this purpose. An article in Annals of The Royal College of Surgeons of England (2008 July; 90(5): 433-434) about a safe support — the "Montreal mattress" — for prone-positioned patients having kidney stones surgically removed through their backs, described the device as "a rectangular mattress with a central hollow which helps prevent compression of the abdomen during respiration." A simple unpatented method is the placement of thick pads, one under the rib cage and shoulders, another under the pelvis, allowing the belly to sag into the space between the pads, minimizing the restriction of breathing. These support measures actually increase pressure on the *chest* with no adverse consequences.

The experience of surgical teams emphasizes several points. First, it shows that such restriction of breathing can occur without any malevolent action. Second, such restriction can occur with only the patient's own body weight compressing the torso, without any external force exerted on the back. Third, because restriction of breathing can be prevented by methods that support the chest and pelvis, allowing the belly to sag into an open space, the mechanism that might otherwise have restricted breathing in these cases is clearly compression of the *abdomen*, not of the *chest*. Fourth, it shows the importance of *anticipating*, based on a person's body type, the likelihood of breathing being restricted by prone positioning, so the person can be handled in a way that *prevents* that restriction. If the police arresting Garner had been adequately trained, they could have similarly anticipated, based on his body type, how seriously his breathing would be restricted by prone restraint on a solid flat surface.

In any case, "chest compression" was a very poor choice of words to convey the proper meaning to the general population. Though most journalists did not explicitly state that the arm around the neck was the cause of chest compression (something the medical examiners could not possibly have been thinking), it seems to be what many journalists thought, since they so often wrote "compression of the neck and chest" without mentioning "prone positioning." An article in the Los Angeles Times (by James Queally and Alana Semuels, Aug. 1, 2014) made that misinterpretation very clear. Their second paragraph began with, "Eric Garner, 43, died after being placed in a chokehold that caused him to suffer neck and chest compressions ...." With "chest compressions" linked to Pantaleo's arm, the "chokehold" was left in most people's minds as the sole cause of death.

Chapter 7

A digression about chokeholds

There are two kinds of chokeholds, differing in their effects, but not looking much different to the untrained eye. One compresses the airway, restricting breathing, and is the one usually just called a chokehold, but sometimes an "air choke." The other chokehold compresses the carotid arteries (and, unavoidably, the jugular veins) on either side of the neck to prevent, or greatly decrease, blood flow through the head and, thus, through the brain. It is most often called a "carotid restraint," less often a "blood choke," and occasionally the very awkward "bilateral vascular restraint."

The carotid restraint, properly (briefly) applied, does not seriously restrict breathing and allows all of the body except the head to remain normally oxygenated, so there is very little decrease of total oxygen in the body. Restriction of blood flow to the brain can render a person unconscious in just a few seconds, but, when the restriction is released, normally oxygenated blood resumes flowing through the brain and recovery can occur fairly quickly. The purpose of this choke is usually to render someone unconscious for a very short time, during which he can be better secured in some other way.

Numerous policemen have described subjecting each other to multiple carotid restraints per day, in their training, and experiencing brief unconsciousness, but no lasting ill effects, so this hold is widely considered safe. However, there are small chances of lasting damage and death. If this kind of choke is weakly applied, the jugular veins, having much thinner walls than arteries, may be greatly restricted, with the carotid arteries inadequately restricted, allowing blood pressure to rise nearer arterial pressure in much of the rest of the cranial circulation. That can cause not just petechial hemorrhages in the eyes, but leakage of blood from capillaries in the brain, resulting in tiny strokes. There is also a chance of dislodging a piece of atherosclerotic plaque, which can move into the brain and cause a very serious stroke. Finally, a phenomenon called a *carotid sinus reflex* might be triggered by this restraint, possibly causing cardiac arrest (though this last effect is still controversial in medical literature and clearly did not happen to Garner, since his heart kept beating long after the alleged chokehold and long after he went unconscious).

In an article on the Breitbart web site, Ben Shapiro asserted that Pantaleo had used a blood choke, rather than an air choke, and that Garner "did not die of asphyxiation." The evidence does not support either of his assertions. First, Garner was conscious and speaking right after the arm around his neck was released, though he should have been unconscious for several seconds after that release if Pantaleo's hold in the preceding eight seconds was actually an effective carotid restraint. Second, the evidence overwhelmingly supports a conclusion that Garner *was* asphyxiated — not by an air choke, but by the prone restraint.

The air choke restricts breathing, depriving the *entire body* of oxygen, and is one of the ways a person can be asphyxiated. This choke takes a considerably longer time than the blood choke does to render someone unconscious, because the brain would only go hypoxic as the entire body goes hypoxic. Therefore, airway compression that is sustained, and probably quite deliberate, is needed to render someone unconscious in this way. When a person has gone unconscious by asphyxiation, the whole body has suffered a very serious loss of its total oxygen. Though resuscitation is possible, it requires a large amount of oxygen to be quickly restored to the body. Attempts at resuscitation after asphyxiation often fail, causing the air choke to be considered more dangerous than the blood choke.

In both kinds of chokeholds, the arm that is directly applying the pressure on the neck is usually grabbed and pulled by the opposite hand to maintain or increase the pressure, meaning that both of the choker's arms are above the shoulders of the person being choked. In the maneuver called a "seatbelt," which is not a chokehold, but a takedown move, neither arm should put pressure on the neck, with one arm pressing down on one shoulder, the other arm pulling up under the opposite armpit, and the arms not necessarily interlocked.

The NYPD instituted a departmental ban on use of chokeholds in 1993. In 1994, Anthony Baez was deemed to have died as a result of a chokehold applied by an NYPD officer. Since then, although there have been several thousand allegations of chokeholds, there has not been another death caused by an NYPD chokehold. We might consider the following explanations for the complete absence of chokehold deaths in that time:

1) Police had learned, and practiced, alternative maneuvers like the "seatbelt" which did not restrict breathing, but which witnesses might interpret as chokeholds.

2) In the process of controlling and restraining a suspect, a policeman's arm may press on a suspect's airway, briefly restricting his breathing, but policemen were trained to adjust their holds as quickly as possible, not doing serious harm.

After the NYPD banned chokeholds, its officers must have been trained in how to avoid or minimize the use of breath-restricting pressure if, during any physical altercation, an officer's arm comes in contact with someone's neck. They might have (and should have) practiced having their arms contact the relatively hard forward projection ("Adam's apple" in men) of the cartilaginous larynx. The only part of the airway accessible to a chokehold is about a three-inch stretch above the collarbones and below the jaw, with the larynx being roughly in the middle of that stretch. An arm that goes into that space, in position to exert significant pressure on the airway, is likely to feel the larynx (though maybe not if the arm is covered by a heavy leather jacket). Officers should have learned to feel the larynx and quickly move their arm to another position if possible, but at least some brief contact with the larynx would be needed for it to be felt. Furthermore, an officer's arm appearing to be on the front of the neck might actually be pressing on the medial ends of the collarbones or up against the chin — acting as a restraint rather than a choke — with the differences not seen by witnesses, but felt by the officer, especially with a bare arm, like Pantaleo's during Garner's arrest.

The evidence of no deaths from NYPD chokeholds since 1994, in spite of the thousands of allegations, suggests that NYPD training has taught its officers that, with physical struggles often proceeding in uncertain ways, possibly including brief movement of an arm over someone's airway, it is most important to avoid sustained choking or damage to the airway.

Chapter 8

The journalists

Quick initial acceptance of the chokehold interpretation of Garner's death concentrated the outrage almost entirely against Officer Pantaleo, with nearly everything he did being reported with the most negative possible interpretation. For example, Pantaleo was holding Garner's head facing to the side during much of the prone restraint, yet many reporters, obviously not studying the video carefully enough, wrote that he was smashing Garner's face into the sidewalk, with some seeming to suggest that this action was restricting Garner's breathing *after* the neck hold had been released. Josh Sanburn quickly wrote

(Time, July 22, 2014), "Orta's video shows what appears to be one officer pressing Garner's face into the sidewalk ...."

Of course, I don't know what was in Pantaleo's mind. No reporters did, either. Yet, nearly all who described this restraint implied malevolent intent on Pantaleo's part. Objective, fair-minded, and adequately observant reporters (what reporters are supposed to be, after all) should at least have *seen* that Garner's head was held with his face to the side and also realized that Garner's words couldn't have been clearly heard if his mouth was against the pavement. Reporters should have considered the *possibility* that Pantaleo intended to keep Garner's mouth and nose unobstructed, along with the *possibility* that NYPD officers were trained to do that.

In TV news reports on Feb. 2, 2018, a video was shown in which Randall Margraves was seen trying to attack Larry Nassar in court during a sentencing procedure. Margraves, a father of girl gymnasts who had been molested by Nassar, was wrestled down in a way that uncannily resembled the takedown and restraint of Eric Garner. One sheriff's deputy reached his arm around Margraves' neck and grabbed his chin, quickly twisting him to the floor, where others joined to hold him in the prone position, pulling his hands behind his back for handcuffing.

During the latter part of the prone restraint, Margraves' head was held with his right ear against the floor, face to his left. Similarly, Garner's head was held with his left ear against the sidewalk, face to his right. Both examples strengthen my impression that many law-enforcement officers are instructed to hold a detainee's head facing to the side during prone restraint, if there are enough hands available for someone to be doing that. This action suggests that currently prevailing warnings about face-down restraint are concentrated on possible obstruction of the mouth and nose, rather than on compression of the torso. People who have been so harshly critical of Pantaleo's holding of Garner's head during the prone restraint need to look at the videos of Margraves' restraint, then re-examine the Orta video.

Margraves was not nearly as hefty as Garner and his prone restraint following the takedown lasted a shorter time, with no signs of him approaching asphyxiation. He was later shown in handcuffs, seated, apologizing to the judge, apparently uninjured by the rough takedown. The takedowns of Margraves and Garner were both "forceful." I think that, knowing the circumstances, virtually everyone considered the takedown of Margraves to be quite proper, since he was clearly "threatening violence" against someone. However, because of Garner's eventual death, the widespread perception of no "good" reason for him to be wrestled down, the failure of almost everyone to understand the later positional asphyxia, and the fact that white officers were arresting a black man, his takedown became described as "brutal, vicious, homicidal violence," even though the evidence indicates that his *takedown*, like that of Margraves, did almost no harm to him.

My first impression, during the broadcast report of the attempted attack on Nassar, was that the deputy pulled on Margraves' *neck*. Later, viewing videos of Margraves' restraint on web sites, I saw that the deputy pulled on Margraves' *chin*. A hand or arm over the airway, even briefly restricting breathing, could actually be safer, since asphyxiating someone with an "air choke" takes a long time, while pulling sideways on the chin may twist the neck, possibly *quickly* causing serious injury to the cervical spine. Thus, there should be some flexibility in judging the propriety of a policeman's actions if his hand or arm goes *temporarily* over the airway of a physically resisting suspect.

Needing to watch more than once to see a hand on the chin instead of on the neck made me more acutely aware that I share with the journalists a common problem of getting things wrong during an initial viewing. Attorneys, judges, and trial analysts are coming to an increasing awareness of the fallibility of witnesses to real-time events, partly because those witnesses lack the ability to "replay" the actual event. However, when the thing we are "witnessing" is a publicly available video, we *can* replay it and — certainly if we are reporters — should take maximum advantage of that ability.

Unfortunately, in the Garner case, it seems that virtually no reporters, or millions of other "witnesses" to the Orta video, reviewed it carefully enough to correct initial misperceptions. They passed on their misperceptions as facts, though I assume not with deliberate dishonesty, but quite possibly with some kind of bias. Such biases might have been, to some extent, pre-existing, but might also have begun with a very emotional reaction to the initial viewing of the video, which just *looked really bad*. Journalists then seemed to lock themselves into their own "echo chamber," repeating or paraphrasing each other's statements, building a shared and *unquestioned* narrative of a chokehold killing.

A day after the Orta video appeared, Police Commissioner Bill Bratton made a statement that included, "... this would appear to have been a chokehold ...." In spite of the tentative nature of *"would appear to,"* that snippet of his statement has been widely represented by reporters ever since then as an *official concession* that Pantaleo *did* use a chokehold. The rest of his statement at that time has been rarely quoted. It continued with, "... but the investigation, both by the district attorney's office as well as by our Internal Affairs, will seek to make that final determination." His qualifying remarks to CNN on Aug. 11, 2014, also rarely quoted, included "... what it appears to be sometimes may not be what it is." Nevertheless, Matt Taibbi asserted, as recently as Nov. 23, 2018 (in Rolling Stone), "The city's police commissioner, William Bratton, conceded Pantaleo had used a banned chokehold procedure."

For some unknown reason, almost all reporters also seemed to make a very early assumption that "prone positioning during physical restraint," was insignificant, though Dr. Sampson's press release put it in the first line of alleged causes of death. An article by Joseph Goldstein and Marc Santora, in the N.Y. Times, began with, "The New York City medical examiner announced on Friday that a Staten Island man died from a chokehold and the compression of his chest by police officers as they arrested him last month for allegedly peddling untaxed cigarettes." Readers had to continue to the *fourteenth* paragraph to find where these reporters finally quoted the words, "and prone positioning during physical restraint," that were actually *between* the words "chest compression" and "by police" in the press release.

Although the prone positioning was sometimes (but far from always) included in other reporters' quotes of that press release, it was almost always left out of descriptions of the arrest. The most common terse description of *what happened* was, as in that L.A. Times article by Queally and Semuels, "Garner died after being placed in a chokehold." This could be called a "sin of omission" on the part of reporters.

Being a scientist, I know how seriously the scientific community views misrepresentation of evidence. Suppose that a scientist does experimental manipulations **A**, **B**, and **C**, in that order, and gets result **D**. If he somehow prefers the idea that **A**, alone, is the cause of **D** and just leaves **B** and **C** out of his research report, that would be a breach of scientific ethics. Try representing the arrest of Garner as such a sequence, with **A** being the takedown, including the alleged chokehold, **B** being the subsequent prone restraint, **C** being the failure of anyone to attempt resuscitation, and **D** being Garner's death. The version of the event most commonly written by reporters was that " **D** followed **A**." Although **D** did come *some time after* **A**, careful study of the total evidence, with knowledgeable interpretation, would reveal that **D** was actually caused by **B** and **C**, with **A** probably being completely irrelevant.

Very commonly, news articles about the arrest of Garner not only omitted the prone positioning, but falsely stated that he was saying, "I can't breathe," when Pantaleo's arm was around his neck. J. David Goodman and Al Baker wrote, in the N.Y. Times, Dec. 3, 2014, "One of the officer's arms went around Mr. Garner's throat, as Mr. Garner repeatedly said, 'I can't breathe, I can't breathe.'"

An NBC New York story (Dec. 4, 2014), said that Garner "is heard saying 'I can't breathe, I can't breathe,' as officer Daniel Pantaleo places him in an apparent chokehold, a tactic prohibited by NYPD policy."

That same day, a USA Today story said Garner "could be heard on a cell phone video shouting, 'I can't breathe,' at least eight times as Pantaleo takes him down in what appears to be a chokehold."

A Boston Globe editorial on Dec. 4, 2014, said that Pantaleo "placed Garner in a chokehold even as the prone suspect rasps repeatedly that he can't breathe."

A CBS/AP story of Dec. 4, 2014, said that the video showed "a white police officer holding the unarmed black man in a chokehold, even as he repeatedly gasped, "I can't breathe."

Jon Sopel, North American Editor, BBC News US & Canada (on Dec. 5, 2014), referred to "the horrible video" and described "... Eric Garner speaking his final words, as this 350 lb giant of a man was held in an apparent chokehold by an NYPD officer."

Months later, in USA TODAY, May 5, 2015, Yamiche Alcindor wrote, "A videotape of the incident shows Pantaleo with his arm around Garner's neck while Garner repeatedly says he can't breathe."

Corinne Segal (PBS web site, July 20, 2015) wrote, after the city reached a financial settlement with Garner's family, "Eric Garner told officers 'I can't breathe' 11 times while in a chokehold by Officer Daniel Pantaleo."

After more than three years, Matt Taibbi still hadn't gotten it right when he wrote in Rolling Stone (Sept. 8, 2017), that "Garner called out, 'I can't breathe' 11 times in a desperate struggle, but officer Pantaleo kept Garner in a chokehold."

Many reporters took it a step further by more directly asserting that the chokehold *caused* the death. The simplest versions of this were, "the deadly chokehold" or "the fatal chokehold," with many of these coming after a grand jury's decision that the evidence did not support even an indictment for a chokehold killing.

Goodman and Baker (N.Y. Times, Dec. 3, 2014) wrote, "A Staten Island grand jury on Wednesday ended the criminal case against a white New York police officer whose chokehold on an unarmed black man led to the man's death."

Eugene Robinson (Washington Post, Dec. 3, 2014) wrote, "The coroner ruled Garner's death a homicide and Pantaleo's chokehold killed him."

In The Guardian, Dec. 3, 2014, Steven W. Thrasher wrote, "Daniel Pantaleo, the police officer who choked Eric Garner to death with a forbidden chokehold, walks free …."

An editorial in the N.Y. Daily News, Dec. 3, 2014, began with, "The grand jury's vote to exonerate the police officer whose chokehold killed Eric Garner on Staten Island has glaring earmarks of a gross miscarriage of justice."

In The Root, on Dec. 5, 2014, David Swerdlick wrote, "Pantaleo had no more legal right to choke Garner to death than a civilian does."

In the N.Y. Times, May 22, 2015, even though this was four months after federal investigators told CNN (Jan. 20, 2015) that they were questioning "whether a chokehold was, in fact, used in restraining Garner," Alexander Burns confidently asserted, "... a police officer's chokehold on Mr. Garner, who was unarmed, led to the man's death."

On Rollingstone.com, July 13, 2015, Simon Vozick-Levinson wrote, "... a grand jury declined even to indict the officer who wrung the life from Garner's neck."

Put the two falsehoods together and you have Chauncey DeVega, on AlterNet, Aug. 13, 2014, writing, "A New York City police officer put his arm around Eric Garner's neck and choked out his life as he gasped, 'I can't breathe.'"

There were many who literally stated that he died *when he was in* a chokehold. Nadine DeNinno, writing in the IB Times, Aug. 1, 2014, began her article with, "The New York City Medical Examiner's Office ruled the death of Eric Garner, the Staten Island man who died in a chokehold by a police officer, a homicide on Friday."

Elahe Izadi wrote, in The Washington Post, Aug. 1, 2014, "The New York City Medical Examiner has classified the death of Eric Garner as a homicide, ruling that the 43-year-old Staten Island man was killed when a police officer put him in a chokehold."

Amy Goodman (on Democracy Now!, PBS, Aug. 25, 2014) reported from a protest march, "This is the site where Eric Garner died in an illegal police chokehold."

An article by Khorri Atkinson in Amsterdam News, on Sept. 25, 2014, was headlined, "Expert pathologist: Eric Garner died in police chokehold."

Beneath the headline, images from the Orta video were captioned, "Eric Garner, innocent father choked to death by NYPD on July 17."

Additional examples came after the grand jury's decision:

Bob Schieffer, who was one of the most respected figures in broadcast journalism, included the following in his opening remark in an interview of Police Commissioner Bratton on Face the Nation (CBS, Dec. 7, 2014): "… outrage following the New York grand jury's decision not to indict officer Daniel Pantaleo after he killed 43-year-old Eric Garner while holding him in a chokehold …."

More than seven months after the grand-jury decision and six months after the federal investigators said that they were questioning "whether a chokehold was used," Corinne Segal flatly stated, on the PBS web site, July 17, 2015, "Eric Garner died in a chokehold by New York Police Department Officer Daniel Pantaleo."

In Time Magazine, July 14, 2015, Sarah Begley wrote, "Garner was killed in a chokehold during an arrest by police on Staten Island."

Even after thirty months, as we were facing the incoming Trump administration and many people felt that a federal investigation into Garner's death would be dropped, Robin Seemangal wrote, in The Observer (Jan. 16, 2017), "NYPD Officer Daniel Pantaleo killed Eric Garner in a chokehold in Staten Island in 2014."

These last four statements were *triply* irresponsible, in that they 1) "convicted Pantaleo in the press," 2) did so *after* the legal process had found that the evidence did not even support indictment for a chokehold killing, and 3) included the blatant falsehood that Garner died *in* a chokehold.

Since the evidence indicates that Garner actually died at least fifteen minutes after release of the alleged chokehold, it is appalling that journalists would twist the evidence in that way. I imagine that journalists might (perhaps with honest intent) excuse this as a *simplification*, saying, "Look, we know the chokehold *caused* his death. What difference does it make if we just say, 'He died *in* a chokehold?'" The difference is that they *only thought they knew* that a chokehold caused his death and the simplification further misrepresented the evidence to support a faulty conclusion even more firmly. It effectively said that no time could have passed between the (alleged) chokehold and his death, thus leaving not even a slim possibility that anything else could have played a role. At least the very common, "He died *after* being placed in a chokehold," though it omitted the most important evidence, left the possibility of an unspecified time span between chokehold and death in which something else, *not mentioned*, might have happened.

Should journalists be excused because two medical examiners seemed to consider a chokehold to be a primary cause of Garner's death? No. According to the autopsy summary, "prone positioning during physical restraint" was also among the primary contributors to his death, but it could not have been a factor if he had *already died in* the "chokehold" that *preceded* the prone restraint. There is no excuse for journalists failing to study the multiple videos, along with other evidence, carefully enough to avoid glaring misrepresentations of what is actually shown.

One extreme example of inept study of evidence combined with strong bias came from Stacey Patton and David J. Leonard on the BBC Viewpoint web site, Dec. 8, 2014:

> Last week a Staten Island grand jury concluded that no crime was committed when an NYPD officer choked 43-year-old Eric Garner to death in broad daylight. Never mind what we all have seen on the video recording; his pleas, and his pronouncement, "I can't breathe."

Had Officer Daniel Pantaleo not choked Eric Garner, the father and husband would be alive today.

Had Officer Pantaleo listened to his pleas, Garner would be alive today.

Had the other four officers interceded, Garner would be alive today.

In America, black lives don't matter because white supremacy requires black death, and it requires that its victims die without sanctuary.

Nothing in this brief article was consistent with the evidence.

1) Since the grand-jury proceedings remain secret, Patton and Leonard did not *know* that the jury concluded that "... an NYPD officer choked 43-year-old Eric Garner to death ...." It seems more likely (though, I admit, also not known) that the jury concluded that Pantaleo's arm around Garner's neck was not the cause of death.

2) If Pantaleo had not even touched Garner's neck during the takedown, but the arrest then continued as seen in the video, with him and the "other officers" all holding Garner in the prone position too long, Garner would have suffered the same deadly positional asphyxia.

3) Ironically, Pantaleo was the one officer who *can* be seen doing something that might have been a response to Garner's pleas — holding Garner's head turned (possibly even according to NYPD training) so his mouth and nose were not directly against the pavement. Unfortunately, that was not helpful because Garner was not experiencing blockage of his airway, but was having his guts crushed up against his diaphragm, something that *none* of the officers there seemed to understand.

4) The final sentence is such a shockingly unsupported leap beyond the *facts of this case* that characterizing Garner's death in this way is light years outside the bounds of responsible journalism.

Another example of journalistic irresponsibility, involving unrelenting, misdirected bias against Pantaleo, misrepresentation of evidence, and blindness to the obvious, was an editorial in the N.Y. Times on Dec. 4, 2014. It deserves to be examined here in its entirety, partly because, although such irresponsibility was seen in the writing of most reporters and commentators dealing with this case, it shows the irresponsibility rising to the top of the field of highly respected news publications. Though I give the Times' editors some credit for publishing one of just two examples I found of writing by professional journalists in which prone restraint was acknowledged to be important in Garner's death, that very acknowledgment made both their outrage at the grand jury's decision and their focused vilification of Pantaleo all the less excusable.

It Wasn't Just the Chokehold

Eric Garner, Daniel Pantaleo and Lethal Police Tactics

By The Editorial Board, Dec. 4, 2014

One route to justice for Eric Garner was blocked on Wednesday, by a Staten Island grand jury's confounding refusal to see anything potentially criminal in the police assault that killed him.

But the quest will continue. The fury that has prompted thousands to protest peacefully across New York City, and the swift promise by the Justice Department of a thorough investigation, may help ensure a just resolution to this tragedy. Mayor Bill de Blasio and Police Commissioner William Bratton, too, have vowed that necessary changes will come from Mr. Garner's death, promising that the Police Department will respond and improve itself, and redouble efforts to patrol communities in fairness and safety.

But among the many needed reforms, there is one simple area that risks being overlooked. Besides the banned chokehold used by Officer Daniel Pantaleo, who brought Mr. Garner down, throwing a beefy arm around his neck, there was lethal danger in the way Mr. Garner was subdued — on his stomach, with a pile of cops on his back.

This breaks a basic rule of safe arrests, especially for people who, like Mr. Garner, are overweight and have medical problems like asthma. When the New York medical examiner's office ruled Mr. Garner's death a homicide, it cited "compression of neck (choke hold), compression of chest and prone positioning during physical restraint by police."

As early as 1995, a Department of Justice bulletin on "positional asphyxia" quoted the New York Police Department's guidelines on preventing deaths in custody. "As soon as the subject is handcuffed, *get him off his stomach*. Turn him on his side or place him in a seated position."

As Michael Baden, a former chief medical examiner of New York City, told The Times: "Obese people especially, lying face down, prone, are unable to breathe when enough pressure is put on their back. The pressure prevents the diaphragm from going up and down, and he can't inhale and exhale."

Which is exactly what Mr. Garner was trying to tell the officers who were on top of him.

Mr. Garner's death recalls a similar tragedy involving a less familiar name: Robert Ethan Saylor, a 26-year-old man with Down syndrome who was killed last year in a struggle with three off-duty county sheriff's deputies at a movie theater in Frederick County, Md. Mr. Saylor was overweight. The officers who killed him were just as inept as Officer Pantaleo and his gang, though with one key difference: When they realized that Mr. Saylor was in distress, they tried to save him. Still, their efforts came too late, because mere moments in a facedown arrest can be deadly.

The Garner killing must lead to major changes in policy, particularly in the use of "broken windows" policing — a strategy in which Officer Pantaleo specialized, according to a report in September by WNYC, which found that he had made hundreds of arrests since joining the force in 2007, leading to at least 259 criminal cases, all but a fraction of those involving petty offenses. The department must find a better way to keep communities safe than aggressively hounding the sellers of loose cigarettes.

And while defenders of the police like to point to thousands of nonfatal misdemeanor arrests as evidence that officers are acting in a way that is reasonable and safe, there can never be a justification for any lethal assault on an unarmed man, no justification for brutality.

The outrage in New York, echoed by anguished protesters in Ferguson, Mo., and in Cleveland, where the Justice Department has found a pattern of excessive force by the police, is based on a genuine fear of aggressive, abusive cops.

The results of such abuse can be seen in the final, quiet minutes of the horrifying video of the Garner assault. This is well after the chokehold, when Mr. Garner lies on the ground as officers and paramedics — who were later disciplined for their behavior — ignore him and bystanders ask: Why is no one giving him CPR?

This was the point where Mr. Garner was dying, the victim of Officer Pantaleo, but also of bad policy, poor training and heedlessness of the basics of anatomy and breathing.

Though the editorial acknowledged the deadly danger of prone restraint, a stubborn acceptance of the chokehold interpretation of Garner's death was so unyielding and the rage against Pantaleo so visceral that the editorial blamed only him by name, from the title to the last sentence.

The editors took their first cheap shot at Pantaleo in the title, essentially making him *the name of* "lethal police tactics."

In the opening sentence, they clearly considered that "justice for Eric Garner" could only be what *they* considered justice — indictment of Pantaleo — rather than the result of the actual legal process, which, in their view, "blocked" justice.

Oddly, the jury's decision was described as a "confounding refusal to see anything potentially criminal in the police assault that killed him." First, there is no evidence that the jury "refused" to see anything. It is most likely that the jury's perception of the Orta video was simply different from the editors' misperception of the video.

Second, the jury was not considering *"anything"* criminal. The DA had granted immunity to all the other officers involved in the deadly prone restraint, so only Pantaleo was being considered for indictment, presumably for something *he alone* did. That should mean that the jury was only considering possible contribution of a chokehold to Garner's death, not the prone restraint that involved the other officers.

Third, what did the editors mean by "the police assault?" If they meant just the takedown, shouldn't they have known that it is proper for someone to be wrestled down if he yanks his arms out of the hands of policemen trying to arrest him? If the editors were including the prone restraint, which they began to describe as lethally dangerous in their third paragraph, did they briefly forget that only Pantaleo was being considered for indictment?

"The banned chokehold used by Officer Pantaleo" continued the condemnation of him in spite of the grand jury's decision, accepting the opinion of two medical examiners as undeniable fact. This might be partly excused, since a statement to CNN by federal investigators that they had begun questioning "whether a chokehold was, in fact, used in restraining Garner" did not come until about six weeks later. Still, the finding of no damage to Garner's airway was reported almost twenty weeks before this editorial, and the video, in which signs of difficulty breathing are detected only during the prone restraint, had also been continuously available for twenty weeks.

The same paragraph has another cheap shot at Pantaleo in the description of his arm as "beefy." Look at the Orta video; there is no visual basis for describing his arm (or even the rest of him) as "beefy." Initially, I saw this as just a *verbal sneer* at Pantaleo, but then began to see it as a way of enhancing the characterization of him as a *brute*, and thus his actions as "brutality."

Then, the editors described the way Garner was eventually restrained as "on his stomach, with a pile of cops on his back." This was an utterly inexcusable falsification of the evidence, since the Orta video does not show *any* cops, much less "a pile of cops," on Garner's back during the prone restraint. The editors may have been misled by Dr. Baden's description of how "obese people especially" are affected by prone restraint, implying that they must have "enough pressure put on their back" to experience deadly asphyxiation. Acceptance of Baden's description might also have led Terry J. Allen to write, in the Jan. 15, 2015, edition of In These Times, that "hundreds of pounds of cop flesh pushed down on" Garner. Possibly partly because of Dr. Baden, but also because of their own woefully careless study of the Orta video, both the Times' editors and Allen *imagined* cops piled on Garner's back to explain his difficulty breathing during the prone restraint. (As previously described, Pantaleo was very briefly on Garner's back when the two rolled over during the takedown, but Garner was on hands and knees then and the deadly compressing of his belly did not begin until his torso was down on the pavement with no cops on his back.)

Later in their lengthy section on prone restraint, although the other officers (not named, of course) were more directly responsible for rolling Garner's torso into the prone position and holding him there too long, the editors still managed another cheap shot at Pantaleo by calling the whole group "Pantaleo and his gang." It was a *double* cheap shot, in that it *named only him* and characterized the group as *"his gang."*

The editors were not yet done with Pantaleo and leveled their most absurd cheap shots at him in the paragraph decrying the "broken windows" crime-fighting policy. They virtually blamed Pantaleo for that policy — again, naming only him. The policy was actually started by Bill Bratton (in his first stint as NYC Police Commissioner) and Mayor Giuliani, about a dozen years before Pantaleo joined the force. The policy continued under Mayor Bloomberg and remained in place when Bratton returned for a second stint as Commissioner under Mayor de Blasio. Matt Taibbi, in his book, *I Can't Breathe*, extensively described the "numbers game" that NYPD officers were forced by their bosses to play, racking up arrests for minor offenses.

Calling broken windows "a strategy in which Officer Pantaleo specialized, according to a report in September by WNYC," the editors grossly misrepresented that report, which actually said that Pantaleo was *not* "specializing" in that strategy, but was just doing what hundreds of other officers were also doing, at the direction of their bosses. That WNYC report by Robert Lewis (Sept. 15, 2014) contained this sequence of three paragraphs about Pantaleo's policing:

"It's clear that he's policing by the numbers," said John Eterno, a former NYPD captain who now runs the graduate criminal justice program at Long Island's Molloy College. Eterno, a critic of the police department's emphasis on statistics, reviewed the records for WNYC.

"This is what the NYPD does," he said. "This is their mainstay. This is their style of policing, at least for the last 12 years. And [for] most officers that are on the NYPD, this is the style of policing that they're familiar with. They know nothing else."

John DeCarlo, an associate professor of criminal justice at John Jay College, also reviewed the records. He said Pantaleo seems to be an average cop and that there were no red flags to indicate a pattern of using excessive force.

Here are two more paragraphs from later in the same report:

Defense attorneys and civil rights lawyers can typically rattle off the names of cops with bad reputations. But a number of attorneys interviewed for this story said they'd never heard of Pantaleo before the Garner case. The Staten Island office of Legal Aid, which provides defense for people who can't afford a private attorney, keeps about 200 files on problem officers in that borough — cops with a history of excessive force complaints or credibility issues. But Pantaleo wasn't one of them.

Pantaleo has been sued twice in federal court for civil rights violations. But court filings show other cops in his precinct have been sued far more frequently.

If anyone in an official position in New York City in 2014 should have been singled out as *responsible for* "broken windows," it was Bratton. Yet, the Times' editors effectively leveled a "backhanded" cheap shot at Pantaleo by *not naming* Bratton in connection with that policy. They only mentioned Bratton earlier, in a positive way, as having "vowed that necessary changes will come from Mr. Garner's death, promising that the Police Department will respond and improve itself."

The complaint about "aggressively hounding the sellers of loose cigarettes" concluding that paragraph was another cheap shot at Pantaleo, since "hounding" means "pursuing relentlessly," but he was reported to be working more serious crimes by 2014, with his assignment to accompany Damico to Tompkinsville Park that day being an exception. It was also a backhanded cheap shot, since Chief Banks, reportedly the driving force behind the intensified crackdown on untaxed cigarette sales in the spring of 2014, was *not named*, leaving Pantaleo the only one implicated by name in this paragraph as "hounding sellers of loose cigarettes."

In the perplexing last two paragraphs, the editors acknowledged that "the point where Mr. Garner was dying" was "well after the chokehold." What happened during the intervening time? The *prone-position restraint!* It was the very thing on which they had spent half their editorial, describing it as possibly quickly deadly, for "obese people especially," even amplifying the danger with the imagined "pile of cops." Having the answer staring them in the face and having actually *put it in their own writing,* they had even less excuse than most other journalists for finding the grand jury's decision so "confounding." They, of all journalists, should have seen that "well after" the alleged chokehold (which *had left no damage to Garner's airway*) it was the prone restraint of Garner by several officers (all but Pantaleo shielded from indictment) that *led to* "the point where Mr. Garner was dying." Yet, stubbornly maintaining their laser-focused condemnation of Pantaleo, the editors took their last cheap shot at him — again naming him alone. In the final sentence, "… Mr. Garner was dying, the victim of Officer Pantaleo ...," was followed, in effect, by "and some other stuff."

The other stuff included "bad policy," apparently referring to "broken windows," for which the street cops actually arresting Garner should not be blamed. It also included "poor training and ignorance of the basics of anatomy and breathing." Since it is obvious that the general population, including most journalists, also lacked enough knowledge of those "basics of anatomy and breathing" to perceive what the Orta video was actually showing, we should not expect such knowledge to have been automatically possessed by the policemen. They needed to get it from their training, which seemed not to have provided it.

This critique of the editorial is not meant to characterize Pantaleo as anything approaching "angelic," but he was no more responsible for Garner's death than were the other officers holding Garner in the prone position for too long. All of them, in turn, might be seen as less responsible than the NYPD that did not train them to understand compressive asphyxia well enough.

After the NYPD started a (slow) process to put Pantaleo through a disciplinary trial for alleged use of a chokehold, an article was placed on the N.Y. Times website (Nov. 7, 2018) with the title, "Eric Garner Died in a Police Chokehold; Why Has the Inquiry Taken So Long?" Those who run the web site strangely ignored their own editors' 2014 description of "the point where Mr. Garner was dying" as being "well after the chokehold."

There were additional examples of journalists strangely twisting evidence to make the officers' actions seem inexcusable. Many reporters described Garner as "raising his hands," but being "assaulted" anyway. Mel Robbins (CNN, Dec. 8, 2014) wrote, "Garner put his hands up, and then one officer grabbed him from behind in a chokehold ...." The wording, "put his hands up," is interpreted by virtually all of us as describing the gesture of *surrender* we commonly recognize, with hands higher than the shoulders, palms forward. In truth, Garner's hands went up that high when he was pulling his arms out of both policemen's efforts to handcuff him. Instead of signaling, "I give up," he was physically resisting arrest.

On Dec. 4, 2014, David Swerdlick (then an associate editor at The Root, more recently assistant editor at the Washington Post) wrote, "I don't consider what Garner was doing 'resisting.' Saying, 'I'm minding my business, please just leave me alone' — which Garner said shortly before Pantaleo jumped him — doesn't sound to me like resisting; it sounds like a Tea Party slogan." How was a reporter/editor so careless (or biased) in his perception of what the Orta video clearly shows that he quoted a statement by Garner, but utterly failed to see the actual *physical* resisting of arrest?

In the same article, Swerdlick bizarrely characterized the takedown of Garner as being done simply because "Garner was huge," adding, "There's no justification for singling out an unarmed man — who's not being violent or threatening violence — for violent treatment, just because he's big." Swerdlick completely missed the point of Garner's size, in terms of how it *should* have affected the way he was handled. The proper point was that police should have been trained to understand how quickly someone of Garner's size and girth could be asphyxiated by prone restraint. On the other hand, the *takedown* of Garner was exactly the opposite of "singling him out," since that is a standard response to *anyone* physically resisting handcuffing during an arrest.

The fact that Garner was "not being violent or threatening violence" was beside the point, but was also mentioned by many other reporters who seemed to be mixing up two different situations:

1) a. You yank your arms out of policemen's hands as they are trying to handcuff you.
   b. They properly wrestle you down to complete the handcuffing.
2) a. You are violently resisting, in ways that may injure the policemen or threaten their lives, possibly with a weapon.
   b. They respond with much stronger force, which they *know* might cause serious injury.

Numerous reporters, like Swerdlick, didn't seem to understand the first situation and wrote reports implying that you must be doing 2a to deserve 1b. The takedown of Garner was a proper response to his resisting of arrest and was not "violent" enough to do any serious harm to him. Unfortunately, the ensuing prone restraint did cause Garner's death, but was not perceived by the police to be deadly while they were doing it, nor recognized as deadly by the vast majority of people, *including journalists*, who mostly ignored "prone positioning during physical restraint" in the autopsy report.

What struck many people, not just reporters, as *apparent* racism, possibly both in the actions of policemen and in the grand-jury decision, contributed greatly to the sense of outrage. Lanre Bakare, an editor at The Guardian, wrote on Dec. 6, 2014, "When a grand jury here in New York failed to find a reason to even send to trial a white police officer who choked the life out of a black man, I finally got it." Of course, if you misinterpret the Orta video as showing a vicious and deliberate chokehold killing of a black man by a white policeman, you would be most likely to see racism both in the killing itself and in the grand jury's decision against criminal indictment. It is, thus, critically important to perceive what journalists as a group failed to perceive — a standard takedown of a physically resisting suspect, followed by the deadly prone restraint, the latter clearly not being a *deliberate* killing, and with neither even being deliberate cruelty.

Statistics do show that about a fourth of those dying at the hands of police are black, though blacks are only about an eighth of the general population, a discrepancy that suggests some involvement of racism. But, those statistics do not show the relative contributions of racism in the minds of policemen versus a much more general socioeconomic unfairness that concentrates blacks in poorer, more crime-ridden areas and leaves some of them financially desperate. The statistics do not justify an *assumption* that the actions of the policemen arresting Garner were driven by racism.

Matt Taibbi's book, *I Can't Breathe: A Killing on Bay Street*, is a special example of reporting on the Garner case, in that it went far beyond the typical short news articles on the topic. It delved into matters well outside the specifics of Garner's deadly arrest, describing his life, the lives of relatives and friends, and his cigarette-smuggling operation, along with a history of racism in the

NYPD and in the nation as a whole, but spent very few words on the actual "killing on Bay Street." In his brief descriptions of those deadly minutes, he seemed to assume that his readers didn't need to be told how Garner died. They could rely on the impressions they had formed during the previous three years from countless news articles and commentaries. He was saying, essentially, "We all *know how* Garner was killed; I'm now showing *the bigger picture*."

Though most of his book is interesting and troubling, reflecting a great deal of research, the research seems to have been entirely peripheral to the specifics of Garner's death. Taibbi had gotten no closer to understanding how Garner actually died. So, on that narrow topic, he simply echoed most of the misconceptions shared by virtually all other journalists, repeatedly calling Pantaleo the killer of Eric Garner, even calling the death "murder" more than once. A year later (in Rolling

Stone, Nov. 23, 2018), Taibbi revealed that he still had learned no more, writing that Garner "was placed in what turned out to be a lethal chokehold."

In the Epilogue of his book, Taibbi wrote that he was "depressed that [Garner] was destined to be remembered only as a political symbol." It is, thus, quite ironic that the whole book was an extended effort to *make* Garner's death political — emblematic of nationwide racism maintained by political leaders. He railed against a DA for miserably "failing" to get an indictment against "Garner's killer" — or "throwing" the case, then "riding it" to a Congressional seat in a Republican-dominated district. He even stretched the case into a factor helping Donald Trump to be elected President.

In his penultimate paragraph he wrote, "Garner's death, and the great distances that were traveled to protect his killer, now stand as testaments to America's pathological desire to avoid equal treatment under the law for its black population." In his penultimate sentence, he described the Garner case as "... about how ethnic resentments can be manipulated politically to leave us vulnerable to the lawless violence of our own government ...."

There is undeniably a long history of racism in this country. It continues to a degree today in spite of some important progress. Opposition to that racism is quite valid. A general case against racist unfairness in our justice system — disproportionately against black *men* — should be amply supported by a great many specific cases and should not require false characterization of the Garner case to support the cause.

In science, we must strive to avoid letting a preconceived notion twist our gathering, presentation, and interpretation of evidence. However, in the

Garner case, it would seem that a desired objective — strengthening a valid case of unfairness against blacks in our justice system and in society at large — twisted the narrative of how Eric Garner was treated on July 17, 2014. Because the truthfully represented evidence in the Garner case does not support an interpretation of racism or brutality on the part of the police officers directly involved, the evidence needed to be egregiously misrepresented to make the Garner case appear to be one of the most glaring and — because of the easily misinterpreted video — *successfully convincing* examples of racist white police brutalizing black men. Most journalists seemed to fall unwittingly into that narrative, probably feeling the rectitude of a greater cause.

Chapter 9

The DA and the grand jury

Virtually the entire population, including reporters, had become that "old-west angry mob," feeling sure of the "chokehold killing" before Dr. Sampson's August 1, 2014, press release, but even more certain afterward, as they focused on that release's initial words and largely ignored the "prone positioning." Most people expected the case to be taken to an ordinary grand jury, which considers many cases in fairly quick succession and which would simply be shown the Orta video, be presented with the medical examiner's findings, and be asked to indict Pantaleo. If the case had been handled that way, an indictment might have been quickly returned, with the whole process taking less than a day. Instead, an "investigative grand jury" was impaneled to consider only this one case, carefully reviewing evidence and testimony to determine if a felony had even been committed and whether a particular suspect should be indicted, a process that ended up taking nine weeks.

Richmond County (Staten Island) DA, Dan Donovan, was reported to have said that he assigned more investigators and attorneys in his office to this case than to any other during his tenure as DA and that his staff began investigating the case immediately after Garner's death. They would then have had more than a month to study the case before Donovan finally announced, on Aug. 19, 2014, that he would "present evidence to a grand jury."

I had needed only three viewings of the Orta video, in less than an hour, to feel convinced that Garner had suffered compressive asphyxia during the prone restraint. It seemed very likely that some of Donovan's investigators knew of the phenomenon they might have called "positional asphyxia." They should also have known, as reported on July 19 and apparently confirmed by the detailed autopsy report on August 1, that no damage had been done to Garner's airway by Pantaleo's arm. Thus, they not only *should* have perceived the *timing problem*, that the arm around the neck could not have directly caused Garner's difficulty breathing during the only time when the evidence shows him having that difficulty, but also should have perceived that the prone restraint, involving several officers, *was* the cause of his asphyxiation.

The lengthy presentation to an *investigative* grand jury after immunity had been granted to the other officers who handled Garner, followed by the jury's decision not to indict Pantaleo, suggested the possibility that Donovan's staff took the case to the jury with the objective of *showing it* that Garner's death was *not* a chokehold killing, while explaining that they considered the deadly prone restraint not to be criminal. It seemed likely that some on his staff knew about the death of Saylor the previous year, resulting in no indictments, and may have known about several cases in Allegheny County, PA, soon described by Harold Hayes in an article posted on Pittsburg station KDKA's web site (Dec. 4, 2014), involving deaths from positional asphyxia during restraint by law-enforcement officers. That story ended with, "None of the local cases mentioned resulted in criminal prosecution of any officer. All resulted in civil settlements." Donovan's staff might also have found, in analyzing training records, that the NYPD officers were not taught an adequate understanding of compressive asphyxia, so indicting them for the prone restraint would be punishing them for being inadequately trained.

While taking a case to a grand jury with the objective of *not* getting an indictment might seem extremely unlikely, it could be consistent with a policy described by Adam S. Kaufmann in the N.Y. Daily News, Dec. 4, 2014. Kaufmann, having been for some years chief of the Investigation Division at the Manhattan District Attorney's Office, wrote, "In my former office, the longstanding policy and practice is to present to a grand jury every case where police action results in a civilian death, whether or not the prosecutors investigating the case think the police conduct was justified. The rationale is that some cases are so important that they must be reviewed by an impartial body — without exception." Thus, if Manhattan prosecutors presented to a grand jury a case in which they felt that evidence did *not* support indictment of a policeman, it would be most ethical for them to present evidence very fully and fairly, with adequate analysis, so the jury might *also* perceive that the evidence did not support indictment.

Many defense attorneys complain that prosecutors virtually always present to grand juries very limited evidence, biased in favor of indictment, so presenting evidence *fairly* in a case against a policeman would be *unfair* to everyone else. Numerous reporters and legal "experts" who were outraged by the grand-jury decision in the Garner case have written that grand juries virtually always vote for indictment when the suspect is not a policeman, but vote against indictment in a significant percentage of cases involving policemen. An extremely important fact that is almost always ignored in this complaint is that prosecutors *do not like to go to trial* with a case they don't think they can win. They tend to be very concerned (probably correctly) that a low conviction rate can stall, or even ruin, their careers, so they may weed out most of the weaker cases themselves. The brief presentation of limited evidence to a grand jury may most often be just a way of speeding the process, rather than an effort to move a weak case to trial.

We should not be surprised that prosecutors almost always get indictments if they usually take to grand juries cases they already think they can win at trial, with possible cases against policemen being a tiny fraction of all the cases they consider. (I concede that prosecutors may consider a moderately weak case against a poverty-stricken member of a racial minority to be "winnable at trial," but consider a similarly weak case against a wealthy white person, or a policeman, to be unwinnable.) If the policy described by Kaufmann, in Manhattan, is followed in cases with a policeman as the suspect, or if a prosecutor feels pressed by intense public outrage to take to a grand jury even weak cases against policemen, we should expect a much lower percentage of indictments in those cases.

It is clear that, in Staten Island, Donovan was not strictly following that "Manhattan" policy, since he granted immunity to the other officers participating in the prone restraint of Garner, leaving Pantaleo the only one who was subject to indictment. The public outcry against Pantaleo was so intense that Donovan might have felt that, at least for Pantaleo, a grand jury was required to decide for or against indictment, with evidence presented very fully and without bias. After the jury's decision, Donovan called the process "a thorough, just and fair investigation." Since the jury could only indict Pantaleo, it could focus on considering whether a deadly chokehold was used, eventually perceiving that Pantaleo's arm was not the cause of death. Donovan's objective might have been to have no policemen put on trial for Garner's death.

Yet, in a report by Murray Weiss in DNAinfo New York, Dec. 16, 2014, (based on unnamed "sources") the DA's attorneys were said to have thought that they presented a convincing case to indict Pantaleo for *criminally negligent homicide*, a felony, and that they "were stunned and disappointed when the panel didn't indict." If the prosecutors had actually tried to get the grand jury to vote *against* indictment *and* if the Weiss story is correct, the prosecutors would have been flat-out lying to Weiss about having *sought* an indictment and I can't go that far down this speculative path.

A somewhat more believable alternative is that Donovan's staff took what may have been the NYC medical examiner's view, that a kind of "one-two punch" caused Garner's asphyxiation, beginning with a chokehold and finishing with the prone restraint, *both* sharing responsibility for Garner's death. If the presentation was thorough and fair, as Donovan eventually asserted, then an explanation of the potential deadliness of "prone positioning during physical restraint" should have been heard by the jury. Since the NYPD had banned chokeholds, but had only advised care in the use of prone restraint and apparently had not trained the officers to understand how someone could be speaking while being asphyxiated, Donovan might have decided that, among the acts that may have contributed to Garner's death, a chokehold was the only one that was potentially criminal, thus the only act for which he could reasonably seek indictment, justifying the immunity he granted the other officers, reportedly in exchange for requiring their testimony to the grand jury (with any perjury invalidating their immunity).

If, as Weiss reported, Donovan's staff honestly thought that their presentation of the evidence had strongly supported indictment of Pantaleo for a chokehold that significantly contributed to Garner's death, the DA's staff must have failed to perceive two things: 1) a complete lack of evidence that there was *any* restriction of Garner's breathing when an arm was touching his neck and 2) the previously described *timing problem* that makes it impossible for that arm to have been limiting Garner's breathing during the only time when the Orta video shows him having difficulty breathing.

The prosecutors might have unwittingly sabotaged their own case by allowing jurors nine weeks to perceive serious flaws in the case. It might have been when Officer Pantaleo testified, reportedly as the last witness, that jurors had their best chance to understand what the Orta video was really showing. J. David Goodman and Michael Wilson (in N.Y. Times, Dec. 3, 2014) wrote, "Officer Pantaleo, 29, led the grand jury through the confrontation, narrating three different videos of the arrest that were taken by bystanders." Those videos lasted only a few minutes each, but Pantaleo was reported to have testified for two hours. That should mean that there was extremely careful, very repetitious, reviewing of video evidence, almost certainly concentrated on the Orta video, which was the only one with the alleged chokehold and the "I can't breathe" statements.

The more carefully the jurors studied the Orta video, the more likely they were to perceive the *timing problem*, with Garner's descent from conscious and speaking to unconscious and limp clearly occurring during the prone restraint, when there was no arm touching his neck and no damage to his airway from the earlier takedown. Such careful studying of the video may have allowed one or more jurors to realize, and then explain to the others, how the evidence simply did not show — even to a standard of "probable cause" — that Pantaleo's arm caused Garner's death, especially if the potential deadliness of prone restraint had already come out in earlier testimony.

How could a prosecutor have failed to see how strongly those two hours of careful study of the Orta video — with Pantaleo's description of what he was doing, and why, at each step — might have affected the jury's view of the case? One possible answer that almost nobody would imagine is that no prosecutor was in the jury room during Pantaleo's testimony. Many prosecutors would react to this suggestion by saying, "That's crazy!"

While I admit that this would be extremely unusual, I have served on a grand jury and know that it is entirely within the power of the jurors to exclude the prosecutor from part, or all, of the testimony of a witness, with the jurors then being the only questioners.

Many legal analysts, writing angrily about the decision of the grand jury in the Garner case, have pointed out that the prosecutors almost always get what they want, as there is no judge or defense attorney present during grand-jury proceedings. However, there *is* a judge involved in impaneling and swearing in the jurors. At that time, jurors are given instructions by the judge, who tells them, among other things, that *they*, not the prosecutors, are legally in charge of the grand-jury proceedings. The prosecutors, in a strictly legal sense, *serve at the jury's behest.* Prosecutors are accustomed to being *effectively* in charge because almost all grand juries just sit back and let the prosecutors "run the show." But, jurors can take charge when they wish and if they understand that they can. It may be something as simple as the jurors wanting to take a few minutes to talk with each other about what they have heard and telling the prosecutor and witness to leave the room when that discussion is taking place, possibly leading to some carefully considered questions the jurors want to pose to the witness after they recall the prosecutor and the witness (or *only* the witness). It can extend to jurors deciding that a particular question asked by a prosecutor is inappropriate and excusing the witness from having to answer that question. For the jury to require the prosecutor to be out of the room during the entire testimony of a particular witness would be more extreme, but legally possible.

One interesting fact about such a situation is that grand-jury secrecy means that even the DA's office does not legally have access to records of what happened in the jury room when no prosecutor was in the room. I have not seen any news reports saying whether there was a prosecutor in the room during those two hours. The story by Goodman and Wilson about Pantaleo's testimony cannot have been based on any direct knowledge of what happened in those secret proceedings and seems to have been based only on what they were told by Pantaleo's attorney. That story did not make a single mention of a prosecutor even being present, much less questioning Pantaleo, and consistently described Pantaleo as talking *to the grand jury*.

I would agree with prosecutors that having no prosecutor in the room during the testimony of a witness would be extremely unusual. However, I face the problem of understanding how a prosecutor present during the jury's very careful review of the Orta video, with Pantaleo's explanations, could have failed to realize how strongly that review affected the jurors' perception of the case.

Numerous critics of the jury's ultimate decision

have asserted that a prosecutor should have torn Pantaleo's testimony apart, showing what the critics called glaring inconsistencies between his "story" (his attorney's version of what Pantaleo said, or was going to say, to the jury) and the critics' descriptions of what they *thought* they had seen in the Orta video. The "inconsistencies" would probably have involved Pantaleo's imperfect memory of the incident (before he testified), critics' misperceptions of the Orta video, or just different interpretations of word meanings. The most commonly mentioned "inconsistency" was that Pantaleo said (according to his attorney) that he "tried to get off Garner as quick as possible," but that the video showed him holding on far longer. What does "get off" mean? The video clearly shows that, *before* Garner started saying, "I can't breathe," Pantaleo *released the neck hold*, just five seconds after Garner was finally brought down onto his right side. The critics, not understanding what Pantaleo was doing *later*, when he was holding Garner's head, may have interpreted *that* as "not getting off."

In any case, the *prior allegations* of inconsistencies would have been irrelevant during Pantaleo's testimony. The only things that would have mattered at that time were the jurors' and Pantaleo's perceptions of what they were all seeing *in the jury room*, as they carefully *and simultaneously* reviewed the video, along with Pantaleo's explanations, *in the jury room*, of what they all saw him doing.

For example, I have a hard time imagining that the jurors would not have wondered why Pantaleo was holding Garner's head the way he was during the prone restraint. The jurors would then, with careful viewing of the video, probably with freeze-frame pauses at critical points, see what so many critics missed — that Garner's head was turned to the side, his left ear against the pavement. (The

Orta video was not nearly as clear as a much sharper video, in 2018, showing the previously described similar holding of Randall Margraves' head turned to the side.) Pantaleo might have told the jury that he learned, in his NYPD training, that someone should try to keep a detainee's head turned to the side during prone restraint, to keep the mouth and nose from being directly on the ground. He might then have told the jury that this positioning of Garner's head, together with the fact that Garner was repeatedly speaking, led him and the other officers to think that Garner *could* breathe. The jury would surely have accepted Pantaleo's description of what the officers all *believed*, even if it realized that the officers were mistaken in that belief. At the same time — especially if a "thorough and fair" presentation had included the deadly danger of prone restraint — they might then have become most strongly convinced that the prone restraint, not the (alleged) chokehold or (disproved) blockage of the mouth and nose, was the likeliest cause of Garner's asphyxiation, with the officers not realizing what they were doing to him.

If there had been a prosecutor in that room, not just seeing and hearing what was going on, but even grilling Pantaleo as harshly as he possibly could, I think he could not have shaken Pantaleo's testimony and should have perceived how seriously the notion of a "deadly chokehold" had been undermined. Therefore, if the Weiss story is correct and the prosecutors were genuinely "stunned" by the jury's decision, I must consider it at least *faintly possible* that no prosecutor was in the room as the jurors carefully reviewed the video evidence with Pantaleo.

The grand jury's decision, on Dec. 3, 2014, not to indict was greeted with nationwide outrage. Journalists commonly called it a "failure." Many politicians and community activists called it "an outrageous miscarriage of justice," as did the previously cited Daily News editorial (Dec. 3, 2014). Trevor Timm, writing in The Guardian, Dec. 4, 2014, called it a "shameful decision by a New York grand jury to refuse to indict the police officer who choked to death an unarmed and unresisting Eric Garner."

The decision was exactly what would have been expected if the evidence had actually been presented very completely, carefully, and without bias, so the decision is not a reason to conclude that there was bias on the part of the jury. But, the decision clashed with journalists' shared misperceptions, which they were completely unwilling to reconsider, so they assumed that the decision resulted from jurors' bias or that jurors had been misled by a conniving DA. Pantaleo continued to be "convicted," both in the press and in the "court" of public opinion.

The original purpose of a grand jury was to protect a person from criminal charges and public trial if allegations were determined to be false or the evidence too weak to justify indictment. A problem with sending someone through a criminal trial resulting in a not-guilty verdict is that such a trial often does not clearly establish innocence. A not-guilty verdict only says that the prosecution did not convince the jury of the defendant's guilt *beyond a reasonable doubt*. Thus, there can remain a widespread public suspicion that the defendant was not actually innocent and that there was *some* justification for putting him on trial. Grand-jury *secrecy* was seen as a way of protecting someone's reputation against spurious charges.

Nevertheless, Randolph McLaughlin, a law professor at Pace Law School, was quoted by Christopher Robbins (in Gothamist News, Dec. 3, 2014) as saying, "Surely they could have indicted this officer on any number of charges and let the public hear, let a trial happen, expose to the light of day what went on here." "Could have," but on what basis? Ignoring the standard of *probable cause* because the angry mob is sure the suspect is guilty? A couple of other lawyers — Lalit Kundani, who had worked as a prosecutor, and Seth Morris, a public defender — expressed a similar view, implying that the grand jury should have been essentially bypassed.

Kundani, in Huffington Post, Dec. 4, 2014, wrote, "The sole function of a grand jury is very limited and minimal. Is there enough evidence to at least justify an arrest in this case? A 'yes' answer does not mean you think the person is guilty. A grand juror can believe a defendant is not guilty of a crime yet still return an indictment." WHAT? For "evidence justifying an arrest" to be enough to send cases to trial would make grand juries just rubber stamps for police departments.

Morris, in an article in the Washington Post, Dec. 8, 2014, wrote, "Probable cause is an exceedingly low standard of proof. All it requires is a *suspicion* that a crime occurred and a suggestion that the defendant *may* be responsible for the crime." (*Italics* were Morris'.) For the grand jury to have a meaningful place in the legal process, it must be able to make a reasonable choice between indicting and not indicting. Although "probable cause" is imprecise and would vary from case to case and from jury to jury, it should not be too close to mere "suspicion" or, at the other extreme, too close to "beyond a reasonable doubt."

Morris ended his article with, "Here's what the right approach should have been: Unarmed men were killed. Let's have a trial." In other words, skip the grand jury and probable cause. Go straight to trial. But, a trial of whom? For doing exactly what? And was the *"what"* a crime? Morris and Kundani, being members of the angry mob, answered those questions, "*Of course* it was Pantaleo. *Of course* it was a deadly chokehold. *Of course* it was a crime." They were just *so sure*, they thought it silly to have a grand jury even consider those questions. At least Morris and Kundani were not saying, "Let's string him up!" But, they were coming close.

Numerous other "legal experts," somehow unable to perceive the obvious *timing problem*, and virtually all without enough knowledge of anatomy and physiology to "see" beyond the visible arm around the neck and understand the invisible deadly squeezing of Garner's belly, offered their opinions based on full acceptance of the chokehold accusation. On the Hugh Hewitt Show (Fox network), legal analyst Judge Andrew Napolitano said it "is clearly a case for criminally negligent homicide."

Law professors Jeffrey Fagan and Bernard E. Harcourt, in a Fact Sheet on the Columbia Law School web site after the grand jury's decision, asked, "Was there probable cause to indict for criminal homicide?" Their one-word answer — by itself as the entire next paragraph — was:

"Yes."

Of all people, law professors working in New York should know that, in New York State, a decision that there *is* probable cause to indict for a felony is made *only* by a grand jury, not by "a coupl'a guys" out there in the general population who *think* they know enough, even if they are law professors. The correct one-word answer to their own question was, "No," because of the decision already made by that grand jury.

Not only did these guys reveal themselves to be quite unable to grasp the importance of the prone restraint, but they thought that the medical examiner's report would stand unchallenged as "probable cause" to indict for a chokehold killing, though they had no knowledge of what the grand jury actually saw and heard, including more careful reviewing of the video. Fagan and Harcourt wrote, "What is clear from the video is that Officer Pantaleo put his arm around Mr. Garner's neck and Mr. Garner stated that he could not breathe while Officer Pantaleo applied neck and chest compression." It is actually clear from the video that *none* of Garner's statements that he couldn't breathe came when an arm was around his neck and that Pantaleo cannot be seen "applying chest compression" at any time.

Far too many, including Fagan and Harcourt, characterized the autopsy report as a "ruling," implying that it could not be challenged. In the justice system, that report would have the status of an *expert opinio*n containing an *allegation* that a chokehold, among other things, played a significant role in Garner's death. For the allegation to lead to an indictment (or eventually a conviction) for a chokehold killing, the medical examiner would still need to appear as a witness attempting to justify the allegation to a jury.

In a HuffPost blog on Dec. 8, 2016, lawyers Joel Cohen and Bennett L. Gershman complained about the grand jury's decision with a sentence that included "... unless the Staten Island Grand Jury that investigated the killing learned something radically different than what the public saw on the clearly incriminating video ...." It is most likely that the jury actually did learn something radically different from what the public (clearly including Cohen and Gershman) *thought it saw* in the not-so-incriminating video.

Many politicians were just as unable to perceive what the Orta video was actually showing about the *physical cause* of Garner's death. Congressional representatives from New York City have been quite outraged, leading to very inflammatory comments.

Rep. Hakeem Jeffries said, "The decision by a grand jury not to indict in the death of Eric Garner is a miscarriage of justice, it's an outrage, it's a disgrace, it's a blow to our democracy, and it should shock the conscience of every single American who cares about justice and fair play."

Rep. Nydia Velazquez said, "I am horrified. Really horrified. How could you sit there as a juror, watch this video and issue a non-indictment?" Unlike Rep. Velazquez, you would at least study the video very carefully, as the grand jury seemed to have done, with the help of the DA's office, and probably with Pantaleo's help during his testimony.

Rep. Gregory Meeks said that the lack of an indictment in Garner's case proved that simply putting cameras on police officers won't solve the problem of abuse of force (reported on HuffPost, Dec. 4, 2014). Meeks' implication was that his interpretation of the Orta video was unquestionably correct, so the "failure" of the grand jury to *agree with him* means that videos can't "solve the problem." Ironically, with some witnesses telling reporters that they saw a chokehold being used on Garner and with a medical examiner finding autopsy evidence seemingly consistent with use of a chokehold, the Orta video is crucial, providing the precise timeline undermining a conclusion that a chokehold caused Garner's death.

Al Baker, J. David Goodman, and Benjamin Mueller (N.Y. Times, June 13, 2015) implied that there was biased manipulation of witnesses, quoting one witness as complaining that the prosecutor told her not to say she saw Garner in a chokehold and not to say he didn't appear to have a pulse just before the ambulance arrived. Preparation of witnesses for testimony can be entirely proper and is actually an ethical responsibility of lawyers bringing witnesses to the stand, either in a trial or before a grand jury. Lawyers are supposed to determine, to the lawyers' satisfaction, that the witnesses really saw what they will be describing in testimony and should advise witnesses to confine their testimony to what they actually saw, not offering conclusions they are not qualified to make. The witness who told reporters she tried to tell the jury that she saw a chokehold and no pulse actually *saw* an arm around Garner's neck and could not possibly have *seen* whether Garner had a pulse. Her *conclusions* that it was a chokehold and that there was no pulse were not proper testimony. In an actual trial, with a defense attorney and a judge present, there would be quick objections. The judge would surely sustain the objections, admonish the witness to stick to what she actually saw, and instruct the jurors to ignore the improper conclusions. However, in grand-jury proceedings, where there is no judge or defense attorney, the prosecutor alone has the ethical responsibility to keep witnesses from veering into their unqualified conclusions or opinions. Though many prosecutors may not be that ethical, it should not be *wrong* for them to be that ethical.

Many journalists and commentators wrote articles characterizing the jury's decision as having to result from jurors' strong initial bias, involving the relatively high percentage of whites living (and thus potential jurors) in Staten Island, along with the fact that many NYPD officers (including Pantaleo) live there. Goodman and Baker (N.Y. Times, Dec. 3, 2014) wrote, "... the jurors deliberated for less than a day before deciding that there was not enough evidence to go forward with charges ...," seeming to imply that their very quick final decision meant that, from the moment they were impaneled, most of them had no intention of indicting a (white) police officer. Such bias cannot be ruled out, but, if the jurors had perceived the *timing problem* and correctly concluded that the evidence did not support any connection between the arm around Garner's neck and his eventual death, they would have needed almost no time in deliberation to decide against indicting Pantaleo for a "chokehold killing," especially if the "thorough and fair" investigation (as asserted by Donovan) had also given the jurors an understanding that prone restraint can be deadly, by itself. Any bias on their part may have just countered the extreme anti-Pantaleo bias in the news every day during the previous four months and enabled them to study the Orta video more open-mindedly to discern what it was actually showing.

Unfortunately, our modern mechanism of spreading gossip — the internet — insured that the allegations against Pantaleo were known all across the country and beyond. Then, the time-honored practice of grand-jury secrecy had the opposite of its originally intended effect. By hiding how the jury's nine-week evaluation of the total evidence might have led to the correct decision not to indict for a chokehold killing, that secrecy left Pantaleo almost universally condemned.

Chapter 10

The Department of Justice

After the Richmond County grand jury's decision, Eric Holder, at that time the U.S. Attorney General, said the Department of Justice would immediately begin its own investigation, under the direction of Loretta Lynch, then U.S. Attorney for the Eastern District of New York, into the possibility that Garner's civil rights had been violated. More than six weeks into that investigation, on Jan. 20, 2015, some of the investigators took a very unusual step of speaking about the case to a pair of CNN reporters, Shimon Prokupecz and Ray Sanchez. Their report quoted the investigators (on promise of anonymity, since the DOJ has a policy against making any public statements on a case still in progress) as saying that they were taking a "fresh look" at the case.

Just on the basis of these two points, journalists should have perked up and taken notice. First, DOJ personnel can be disciplined, perhaps up to being fired, for unauthorized revelations, so they should have been seen as having a very strong motivation for saying *anything* to the press at that time. Second, the words "fresh look" should have suggested to perceptive journalists that the case handed to the DOJ in the first week of December, seemingly a vicious chokehold killing that resulted in no criminal indictment at the state level, was looking like something different to the feds after six weeks of their own analysis.

Nestled among the investigators' other, rather innocuous, remarks was one that should have had all journalists slapping themselves on the forehead and yelling, "WHAT?!!" It was that the "fresh look" included questioning "... whether a chokehold was, in fact, used in restraining Garner." If the feds still believed that the arm around the neck was the cause of death, they would have *had to* consider it a chokehold. Journalists should have asked themselves, "How could the arm around the neck NOT have been a chokehold if it KILLED him?!"

"How could it not have been a chokehold if it..."

"Oh..."

"Hmmmm..."

How could the feds have wondered whether the arm around the neck even *was* a chokehold without perceiving *at least* that it was not *obviously* the cause of death? Yet, it would seem that not one journalist in the world perceived that implication. Even Prokupecz and Sanchez seemed to ignore it, since the opening sentence of their CNN article described the incident as a "chokehold death of an unarmed black man at the hands of a white police officer."

Were the feds trying to reveal, in a very carefully oblique way, that they had realized what might have led the Richmond County grand jury to vote against indictment — that the evidence pointed toward deadly positional asphyxiation? The feds may have been walking a narrow line, trying to protect their jobs while *just nudging* journalists to consider the possibility that Garner's death could have been caused by something other than a chokehold.

Journalists were not nudged.

If the investigators had determined that the arm around the neck was not the cause of death, why would they even be wondering if it was, "in fact," a chokehold? You might recall the beating of Rodney King during an arrest in Los Angeles in 1991. Federal charges were brought against policemen involved, with two being convicted of violating King's civil rights by using excessive, unwarranted force against him. King suffered serious injuries, including a fractured skull, from the beating with clubs ("batons"), but he survived and lived another 21 years. The important point, with regard to the Garner case, is that the excessive force need not be fatal to be a violation of civil rights. Thus, even if Pantaleo's arm around Garner's neck had not caused Garner's death, there was still a slim possibility that, if it had been "in fact" a chokehold, banned by the NYPD, Pantaleo might have been charged at the federal level with violating Garner's civil rights by *intentionally* using *excessive, unwarranted* force.

That would be a difficult case to make for multiple reasons, including a need to show *intent* to do harm. The federal requirement of intent is sometimes met by a determination that virtually anyone in the general population would understand that a particular action can cause serious injury, but the person being considered for indictment did it anyway. Beating someone with a club, as in the Rodney King incident, would meet that criterion.

In contrast, as made very clear by the reactions of reporters and the general population to the Orta video, almost nobody understood the deadly danger of prone restraint, so that action would not meet the same criterion. However, a chokehold might, especially if it could be shown to have been, "in fact," a chokehold.

The federal investigators were surely knowledgeable enough about chokeholds to perceive very quickly that the way Pantaleo first tried to take Garner down — right arm under right armpit, left arm over left shoulder — was obviously not any kind of "choke" hold, meaning that Pantaleo did not initially demonstrate either the required *intent* to choke Garner or a *reasonable knowledge* that whatever he was doing had *any potential* to cause great harm. Second, the investigators would not have been able to find clear evidence that there was *any* restriction of Garner's breathing when the arm was around his neck, before he was rolled into the prone position. Third, compared to King's serious injuries, the only injuries to Garner that can be clearly attributed to an arm against his neck were slight enough not even to be noticed during external examination. If the subsequent deadly positional asphyxiation had not led to an autopsy, the bruising of neck muscles would not have been detected at all and thus would be difficult to characterize as caused by *excessive* force. Fourth, even those injuries were not directly to any part of the airway, but to muscles on either side of the airway. Fifth, since Garner had clearly resisted arrest, the degree of force used to bring him down with such minimal injury could hardly be considered *unwarranted*.

The immunity granted by Donovan to the other NYPD officers applied only to state charges, so federal charges could have been considered against the whole group involved in the prone restraint (including Pantaleo), if the feds had perceived that restraint to have been the actual cause of Garner's asphyxiation. Here, *intent* would have been an even greater hurdle for the feds, since prone restraint is neither banned by the NYPD nor considered, in most cases, to be excessive or cruel and is very widely used by police around the country. If the feds considered such charges, they were likely to have determined that the NYPD officers were not taught an adequate understanding of compressive asphyxia, so "intent to do harm" with this restraint would have been virtually impossible to establish. Furthermore, if the DOJ had previously looked into other cases involving deadly positional asphyxia without deciding to indict, then their own precedent should have weighed heavily against criminal indictments for the deadly prone restraint of Garner.

The DOJ would almost certainly have also looked for evidence of racist motivation on the part of officers handling Garner, since that would have been another way Garner's civil rights could have been violated. The mere fact that Garner was black, while the two officers initially placing him under arrest were white, would not be seen as evidence of racism (though there were millions in the general population who felt that it was). Consider the remote possibility that there was no racism in the hiring of police officers throughout the nation and no differences in the desires or qualifications of people in different ethnic groups to become police officers. Then, the fraction of all police who are black would reflect their fraction of the total population — about one eighth. The probability that a single arresting officer is not black would be $7/8$, over 87%. If there were no racism in policing policies and two officers were arresting a black man, the probability of neither officer being black would be $7/8 \times 7/8$, about 77%. Thus, though we don't have that ideally unbiased situation, the fact that two officers arresting Garner were not black could be consistent with the numerical odds and the feds would need clear evidence of *racist motivation* behind the actions of the officers directly handling Garner to charge them with a racist violation of civil rights.

Many people viewing the Orta video quickly assumed that the incident involved a couple of white officers cruising around, looking for a black man to harass, picking on him for a minor offense, then treating him as they would never treat a white man. There is ample evidence that a great many young black and Hispanic men in New York City have been subjected to that kind of harassment under the policies called "broken windows" and "stop and frisk." However, in any single case, the feds would need to use *evidence in that case* as the basis to prosecute for racism. In this case, they should have learned that Chief Banks, himself a black man, had ramped up the campaign against sellers of smuggled cigarettes just before Garner's deadly arrest and that the officers who arrested

Garner were sent by their superiors to *that* location at *that* time to deal with *that* specific "problem." Furthermore, white men who similarly resist arrest are also typically subjected to forcible takedown and prone positioning. Since the initial group of DOJ investigators and attorneys did not see a basis for *any* indictments of the officers handling Garner, they must not have seen evidence of racism behind the actions of those officers.

There is still, in this country, some pervasive socioeconomic unfairness against blacks, the residue of generations of much worse unfairness — slavery, Jim Crow, and legal segregation. Although things have gradually improved, the lingering effects of that more extreme unfairness keep some people experiencing poorer housing, jobs, and education, along with neighborhoods that make it difficult for growing children to imagine better opportunities for themselves. Legal rulings of unconstitutional "reverse discrimination" have blunted many efforts to alleviate those problems.

Even quite recently, poor people have been deliberately tricked by financial institutions and real-estate developers. Blacks were hurt much worse than whites by the 2008 financial crash and the ensuing deep recession. With the election of Donald Trump, many previously hidden racists have "come out of the woodwork," showing that we have far to go to get fully beyond racism.

There remain instances of racist unfairness at all stages within the justice system, including initial encounters with police, subsequent interrogations, decisions of prosecutors, quality of legal representation, jurors' biases, and sentencing decisions. For decades, an extremely unfair legal distinction between crack cocaine and powdered cocaine caused the ratio of blacks to whites in prison for drug offenses to be much higher than the ratio of blacks to whites actually using or selling illegal drugs, resulting in a disproportionately large number of broken black families, with black men struggling to succeed after release from prison.

Non-whites facing a pervasive unfairness are more likely to slip into what is sometimes called the "gray economy" or "underground economy," involving work that is not completely in compliance with all laws. That makes non-whites more likely to be caught up in the "broken windows" emphasis on minor offenses in New York City. Although the diffuse and pervasive unfairness *is* lingering racism, it does not constitute the sort of direct, specific racism for which federal prosecutors could seek indictments of the officers arresting Garner.

The DOJ's continuing problem with reaching a resolution of this case is troubling. The failure of the initial group of DOJ investigators and attorneys to convince their colleagues in Washington, DC, not to seek indictments on federal charges, together with the Weiss story about the Richmond County prosecutors being "stunned" by a grand jury's decision not to indict, would suggest that neither group of prosecutors adequately perceived *both* the overwhelming evidence pointing to compressive asphyxia by prone restraint *and* the paucity of evidence that the arm around the neck played any role in Garner's death.

The initial group of DOJ investigators may not have argued that the arm around the neck did almost no harm, just that a *lack of intent to do harm* extended through the 15-second takedown, while attorneys in the DOJ Civil Rights Division felt that the neck hold *became* willful wrongdoing when it was not released quickly enough after Garner was pulled down, even if they can't show that it did *any* harm during those additional seconds. The decision of the initial DOJ investigators against indictment was ultimately rejected in 2016 by Loretta Lynch, who replaced Eric Holder as Attorney General on April 27, 2015.

When those DOJ Civil Rights attorneys recently asked Dep. Attorney General Rod Rosenstein to renew an effort to indict Pantaleo, Matt Apuzzo, without directly quoting anyone, wrote (N.Y. Times, April 20, 2018) that the civil rights prosecutors "… said the video, captured by a bystander, showed clear evidence of willful wrongdoing. In particular, they have singled out the moments after Officer Pantaleo was clear of the storefront window and appeared to keep putting pressure on Mr. Garner's neck." In the same article, Apuzzo wrote, "… civil rights prosecutors said it represented a clear case of excessive force."

Determination that force is excessive should usually depend more on the *degree of harm* than on the *duration* of a particular action. Just one blow to the head with a club, fracturing the skull, could easily be deemed excessive, even though the force lasted only a fraction of a second, while force used to maintain restraint of a resisting suspect even for several minutes might not be deemed excessive if it only caused some bruising. Since Pantaleo's sharp yank of Garner away from the storefront window might reasonably be seen as the moment when he applied the strongest force — force that the DOJ attorneys, themselves, seem to consider justified by the imminent danger of broken glass — that moment may be argued to be when neck bruising was most likely to have occurred, with Pantaleo's arms not then in the position of a chokehold. Prosecutors would be unable to show a trial jury that any bruising occurred later and would be unable to show evidence of *any* restriction of Garner's breathing during the entire fifteen seconds from the start of the "seatbelt" until the release of the neck hold. So, how could the *five seconds* from the time Garner finally came down on his right side (ending his resistance) to the time Pantaleo's left arm came off Garner's neck have constituted "excessive force," since Pantaleo might reasonably have taken those few seconds to assure himself that the other officers had gained adequate control and to extend his own right hand to grasp Garner's right wrist? If those Civil Rights prosecutors consider Pantaleo's later holding of Garner's head during the prone restraint to be part of Pantaleo's continued "pressure on Mr. Garner's neck," rather than a turning of Garner's head to keep his face unobstructed, their inept study of the evidence would be very troubling, since the DOJ had more than three years to examine the Orta video.

Attorneys in the Civil Rights Division may not be much different from the many civil-rights attorneys outside government who were among the people most strongly critical both of the handling of Garner during the arrest and of the eventual decision by the Richmond County grand jury. The Civil Rights Division may also have been strongly influenced by intense pressure from politicians in DC, described by Mike Lillis in The Hill, Jan. 12, 2017, perhaps mainly from New York City congressional representatives, who have been unrelenting in their insistence that the "chokehold killer" *must* be punished in some way.

My strong suspicion is that most civil-rights attorneys have continued to believe that Garner's arrest was not only a chokehold killing, but a particularly glaring example of *racist* policing, a belief expressed in a commentary (on msnbc.com, August 5, 2014) by Judith Browne Dianis, a civil-rights attorney and co-director of the Advancement Project in Washington, DC. When I belatedly found her article, its title, "Eric Garner was killed by more than just a chokehold," suggested that one more rare person might have perceived the importance of "prone positioning." Instead, the article asserted that "implicit bias" was the other thing that killed Garner, with agreement from Donna Lieberman (NYCLU) who said that the way Garner was handled "would never happen to a white person."

Dianis described Garner as "catching the eye of the police" simply because he was seen "breaking up a fight," not because the police had seen him committing even a minor crime. She then wrote, "Garner wanted to know why he was being harassed, and he paid for that query with his life. In America, we're not supposed to kill people for questioning an officer." Essentially, her extreme twisting of the evidence was that Garner was *killed* for being a black man who had the temerity to talk back to white policemen.

However, attorneys in the Civil Rights Division, like the initial DOJ investigators, would not be able to *show* that the officers arresting Garner either lacked any justification for arresting him in the first place or would have handled a white man any differently if that man *physically* resisted arrest exactly as Garner did. So, with indictment for racist violation of civil rights probably out of reach, indictment for use of excessive force seemed a more realistic possibility. Since so many civil-rights activists feel that the DOJ is the last chance for anything like the "justice" they have been demanding in the Garner case, many attorneys in the Civil Rights Division must feel that they can't let this case slip away without *any* indictments. Pantaleo is the obvious target, since most people, including journalists, still mistakenly believe that he choked Garner to death.

Dep. AG Rod Rosenstein was reported to be against the indictment, considering the case to be "unwinnable" at trial, possibly partly because any of the original DOJ investigators and attorneys who decided against indictment could be called as witnesses *for the defense.* If Rosenstein and then-AG Jeff Sessions had perceived just how weak the evidence against Pantaleo really is, they should have rejected indictment much earlier (as Loretta Lynch should have done in 2015), confident that they could justify that decision. The ongoing disagreement within the DOJ suggests that *nobody* in the DOJ has fully understood what the evidence — especially the Orta video — really shows.

Now, a new AG and, perhaps soon, a new Dep. AG, possibly having too little knowledge of the case, could decide just to drop it (the statute of limitations prevents indictment after July 17, 2019), or they could yield to lawyers in the Civil Rights Division, whom they might consider to have a better grasp of the case. So, there is still a possibility that we will end up seeing a strange situation in which the actions that actually caused Garner's death — his prone restraint by several officers — result in no indictments at any level of government (though reasonably, since those actions seem to have resulted from poor training), while one policeman *does* get indicted for doing something that *looked bad*, but which neither killed nor even seriously hurt Garner.

In my opinion, a proper outcome of the federal case would be no indictments of the policemen directly involved in Garner's arrest, a publicized analysis of what really happened in that incident, and a strong directive that a more complete understanding of "restraint-related positional asphyxia" be taught to all law-enforcement officers throughout the country as quickly as possible. Unfortunately, conflicting factions within the DOJ still need to discern, with more thorough and knowledgeable analysis of the evidence, what *actually happened.*

Chapter 11

The CCRB and the NYPD

Though the federal case may be concluded with no indictments of any policemen involved in Garner's arrest, there is going to be an NYPD disciplinary trial of Officer Pantaleo, the severest penalty probably being termination of employment by the NYPD. In a preliminary hearing on Dec. 6, 2018, that trial was set to start on May 13, 2019.

According to Matt Taibbi (Rolling Stone, Sept. 8, 2017), New York City's Civilian Complaint Review Board "ruled that Pantaleo did in fact use a chokehold, and also ruled that Pantaleo restricted Garner's breathing." The CCRB's decisions were *not* "rulings." One needed to read much farther in

Taibbi's article to find where he wrote, "The CCRB ... merely investigates abuse allegations against police and issues recommendations for or against internal police discipline. CCRB findings are forwarded to the Police Commissioner and to the city's Department Advocate's Office, who ultimately issue disciplinary rulings." Oh, *that's* where "rulings" come.

In his initial sentence, Taibbi said that the Board "substantiated two allegations against Daniel Pantaleo," with the word "substantiates" also in the article's title. Because the Board's report is still confidential, we only have brief descriptions, from unnamed "sources," of those two allegations and no revelation of any evidence that the Board considered to "substantiate" the allegations.

Definitions of the word "substantiate" in various dictionaries include "verify," "provide evidence to support or prove the truth of," "show something to be true," and "support a claim with facts."

According to numerous reports, the Board just uses the word "substantiated" to label the category of complaints having what it considers the highest believability, without necessarily "substantiating" them according to the dictionary definitions. By those definitions, the Board would be unable to *substantiate* a conclusion that Pantaleo's arm around Garner's neck actually restricted breathing. Without access to the secret report, we don't know if the Board also thought that Pantaleo was restricting Garner's breathing by holding Garner's head during the prone restraint, something they would also be unable to substantiate — except to the extent that he was one of several officers holding Garner down on the sidewalk. Since the Board has not leveled charges against the other officers who were restraining Garner, its charge that Pantaleo restricted Garner's breathing must be based only on the alleged chokehold.

The Board's decision that Pantaleo used an NYPD-banned chokehold might have been made easier by the NYPD patrol guide's very fuzzy definition of "chokehold," which contains (with my italics) the odd wording, "including, *but not limited to*, a hold that exerts *any* pressure to the throat or windpipe, which *may* prevent or hinder breathing or reduce intake of air." However, a 2015 report, "Observations on Accountability and Transparency in Ten Chokehold Cases," by the NYPD's Office of the Inspector General, contained the sentence, "The CCRB tended to substantiate cases based specifically on whether credible evidence indicated contact between the subject officer and the complainant's neck in a manner that interfered with breathing." I strongly suspect that the initial DOJ investigators also felt that they needed to see *evidence* that Pantaleo's arm actually restricted Garner's breathing for them to consider that a chokehold was ("in fact") used on Garner and could find no such evidence. The departmental trial should reveal what the CCRB considers evidence supporting a *charge* that Pantaleo's arm *did* restrict Garner's breathing.

Anticipating that trial, the NYC Patrolmen's Benevolent Association released a statement quoted by Richard Khavkine in The Chief Leader, Dec. 10, 2018, that the full autopsy report "demonstrates conclusively that Mr. Garner did not die of strangulation of the neck from a chokehold." In an article on timesunion.com, by Michael R. Sisak (Associated Press), the PBA statement was said (without quotation marks) to have indicated that Garner couldn't have been subjected to a chokehold because the autopsy showed that his windpipe and hyoid bone were intact. Dr. Sampson was quoted by Sisak as offering the rebuttal, "It is false that crushing of the windpipe and fracture of the hyoid bone would necessarily be seen at autopsy as the result of a chokehold." While that is true, the lack of damage to Garner's airway would *also* be consistent with him *not* being subjected to a chokehold, requiring other evidence to support a *charge* that he was choked. The total evidence does not support a *conclusion* that Garner was choked by Pantaleo's arm because the *video* shows all evidence of difficulty breathing coming after the arm was released and the *autopsy* shows that the arm left no damage to the airway to restrict breathing after release of the arm. Though we cannot completely rule out some *unnoticed* brief restriction of breathing when the arm was in contact with Garner's neck, the evidence strongly supports the statement that "Mr. Garner did not die of strangulation of the neck from a chokehold."

In AM New York (Sept. 11, 2017), Len Levitt wrote, "The Civilian Complaint Review Board ... has determined Pantaleo applied a department-banned chokehold on Garner, killing him." Those last two words, "killing him," had to spring from

Levitt's own highly biased imagination. I have not seen them in any other published description of what the CCRB decided. Though some CCRB members may believe that choking by Pantaleo made a significant contribution to Garner's death, their report should be limited to charges that would fall under a departmental disciplinary process, with criminal homicide charges only pursued under state law. Whatever Levitt might have guessed that CCRB members *personally believed*, it was inexcusable for him to attribute those two words to the unpublicized CCRB charges.

Levitt's article went much further, stating, "That the CCRB has stepped in is an implicit sign that traditional law enforcement agencies — a district attorney's office, the Justice Department and the NYPD — have made the case a mockery of justice." It is actually an enormous "angry mob," including journalists, that has made the case a mockery of justice. Completely outside the legal system, members of that mob have "convicted" a policeman of a chokehold killing because they didn't study the evidence carefully enough, didn't know important parts of the total evidence, or didn't possess the necessary knowledge to interpret the evidence correctly. They simply jumped to their own conclusions, which they were then completely unwilling to reconsider when the legal process didn't deliver the result they wanted. Most of the very few people who actually studied the evidence carefully, and came at least closer to interpreting it correctly, seemed to be in the Richmond County special grand jury in 2014 and in the DOJ's Eastern District of New York in 2015. Unfortunately for us, they were blocked by law or by departmental policy from explaining their findings to the public (or to the CCRB).

The NYPD has a record of greatly reducing the CCRB's recommended penalties against officers, but the NYPD may face a serious problem if the DOJ decides against indicting Pantaleo *without explanation*. Many NYPD officers who were alleged to have used a chokehold in the years since the NYPD's banning of chokeholds have received little or no departmental punishment. Since Pantaleo's arm around Garner's neck was never established in court to have done any more harm than alleged chokeholds by those other officers (or even to have *been* a chokehold), how would the NYPD justify treating Pantaleo completely differently? Conversely, how could the NYPD keep Pantaleo on the force if he continues to be so demonized by almost everyone in the entire population? Could it ever put him back on the streets without surrounding him with protection? Would Pantaleo have to be "thrown under the bus" for the sake of better public relations?

The answers would probably depend on how well the misconceptions held by almost everyone can be corrected. If the DOJ decides — properly — not to indict any policemen involved in Garner's arrest, the DOJ needs to be able to explain very fully, in its final report, what it perceived the policemen to have done during Garner's arrest. If the DOJ can come to an internal agreement that Garner's death resulted not from a chokehold, but from the extended prone restraint, that the latter was done by several officers who had not been trained by the NYPD to have an adequate understanding of compressive asphyxia, and that they did it without *intent* to do harm, the DOJ should make that clear.

The Police Commissioner — regardless of the judge's decision in the upcoming departmental trial — should reject the CCRB's misguided recommendation of severest disciplinary action against Pantaleo, and should issue a major *mea culpa*, conceding the NYPD's failure to train the officers well enough. Responsibility for the NYPD training program rises specifically to the level of one of the Deputy Police Commissioners and it would be unjust for street cops to be punished because the faulty training led to a death.

Postscript

I have been strongly critical of journalists' handling of the Eric Garner case and consider that criticism to be well justified. However, I hope that the vast majority of reporters working in what we call the "mainstream news media" have a conscious desire to be responsible, ethical journalists. (The "tabloids" and the right-wing commentators are a lost cause.) I would hope to be able to rely on most "mainstream" news reports to be carefully checked and factually correct. Those journalists with the honest intent to be responsible may have been just thrown off by certain characteristics of the Garner case.

"Smart-phone" videos of people's encounters with police are a relatively new phenomenon, with

Ramsey Orta's video giving millions of people, including virtually all journalists, a sense that they saw all that they needed to see in order to understand exactly what happened. Numerous journalists described the Orta video as being "crystal clear" and leaving "no doubt" about what happened. What they *concluded* from viewing the video was mistakenly considered to be what it *clearly showed*.

With the video not literally *showing* what was happening inside Garner's torso, journalists locked in on the visible "chokehold," unquestioningly accepting the initial words in Dr. Sampson's press release, but almost completely ignoring the "prone positioning," which the ME did not specifically state to be less important than "neck compression."

In addition, a very emotional response seemed to come from viewing the video with advance knowledge that Garner's death was the outcome. Emotion is not to be disparaged and may often serve as a strong motivator to pursue a story and "get the truth out." Unfortunately, in this case, the emotion seemed to drive reporters to a degree of outrage that interfered with their ability to be unbiased, possibly keeping them from reviewing that very troubling video and studying it carefully enough even to describe it accurately, much less to interpret it correctly.

The modern phenomenon of the internet, with its "blogs," Twitter, and readers' rapid responses appended to web pages of news stories, has put reporters in an unfamiliar position of being vulnerable to being quickly swept along with the opinions of millions of people, feeling comfortable with the nearly unanimous support for a particular viewpoint, and perhaps even being subconsciously swayed to hold that viewpoint before writing their own reports.

I am aware of the modern problem of people abandoning subscriptions to traditional newspapers in favor of getting, at no cost, what they hope are reliable news reports on the internet. Loss of income for print journalism has limited the amount of thorough research that can be done, in this case seeming to cause reporters to do a great deal of echoing of other reporters' statements. Still, how difficult is it to sit down at a computer, open a web browser, and type in the words from the medical examiner's press release, "prone positioning during physical restraint," to find explanations of the deadly danger of that restraint, especially for someone who is obese, then to wonder if that *could* have been a factor in the grand jury's decision?

Reporters seemed to sit back and wait for a very unlikely release of records of the grand jury proceedings, as if thinking, "We can't do anything until we know what went on in the jury room." Actually, all the evidence needed for reporters to figure out why a police officer would not be indicted for a chokehold killing was available to the general public, mainly in the form of that poorly studied video. Reporters needed to free themselves from their hastily solidified view of the case and study the available evidence more carefully and open-mindedly.

I also had the impression that most reporters felt a need to be on the "right side" of an important social issue — standing for fairer treatment of blacks in the justice system. However, for reporters, supporting a valid larger cause should never be inconsistent with adhering to professional responsibilities and ethics in covering a specific case.

It is my hope that journalists will not simply have an angrily defensive reaction to this book, but will take a good look in the mirror, perceive how badly they went wrong in covering the Garner case, and resolve to make very conscious efforts to avoid falling into the same traps in the future.

www.ingramcontent.com/pod-product-compliance
Lightning Source LLC
Chambersburg PA
CBHW070936180526
45158CB00023B/1384